ADVANCES IN ANIMAL WELFARE SCIENCE
1984

ADVANCES IN ANIMAL WELFARE SCIENCE 1984

edited by

Michael W. Fox, D.Sc., Ph.D., B.Vet.Med., MRCVS
Director, The Institute for the Study of Animal Problems
Washington, DC 20037, USA

and

Linda D. Mickley B.S.
Research Associate, The Institute for the Study of Animal Problems
Washington DC 20037, USA

1985 **MARTINUS NIJHOFF PUBLISHERS**
a member of the KLUWER ACADEMIC PUBLISHERS GROUP
BOSTON / DORDRECHT / LANCASTER

Distributors

for the United States and Canada: Kluwer Academic Publishers, 190 Old Derby Street, Hingham, MA 02043, USA
for the UK and Ireland: Kluwer Academic Publishers, MTP Press Limited, Falcon House, Queen Square, Lancaster LA1 1RN, UK
for all other countries: Kluwer Academic Publishers Group, Distribution Center, P.O. Box 322, 3300 AH Dordrecht, The Netherlands

Library of Congress Cataloging in Publication Data

ISBN 0-89838-699-3

PRINTED IN THE NETHERLANDS

MANUSCRIPT REVIEW COMMITTEE ADVANCES IN ANIMAL WELFARE SCIENCE

B. O. Hughes	Agricultural Poultry Research Centre, Roslin, Midlothian, Scotland
Frank Hurnik	Department of Animal Science, University of Guelph, Guelph, Canada
Ron Kilgour	Ministry of Agriculture and Fisheries, Ruakura Animal Research Station, Hamilton, New Zealand
Devra Kleiman	National Zoological Park, Smithsonian Institution, Washington, D.C., USA
Elizabeth A. Lawrence	Tufts University, School of Veterinary Medicine, Boston, Massachusetts, USA
Michael J. McCulloch	Northwest Resource Group of Mental Health, Portland, Oregon, USA
Jenny Remfry	Universities Federation for Animal Welfare, Potters Bar, Herts, England
Bernard E. Rollin	Department of Philosophy, Colorado State University, Fort Collins, Colorado, USA
Andrew N. Rowan	Tufts University, School of Veterinary Medicine, Boston, Massachusetts, USA
Harry C. Rowsell	Canadian Council on Animal Care, Ottawa, Ontario, Canada
Joyce S. A. Tischler	Attorneys for Animal Rights, San Anselmo, California, USA
G. van Putten	Research Institute for Animal Production, "Schoonoord", Zeist, Holland
D. B. Wilkins	Royal Society for the Prevention of Cruelty to Animals, The Causeway, Horsham, Sussex, England
Thomas Wolfle	National Institutes of Health, Department of Health and Human Services, Bethesda, Maryland, USA

EDITORS' FOREWORD

This book, the first in an annual series, written by academicians—scientists, philosophers and others—is not intended exclusively for animal welfarists and conservationists. Since it is written* by scholars, it will appeal to a wide range of academic and professional readers who are involved with animals for scientific, economic, altruistic, and other reasons. While this first volume cannot cover the entire spectrum of animal welfare science-related topics, it does, in its diversity of contributions, demonstrate the multi-faceted and interdisciplinary nature of the subject of this new series.

Indeed, animals are as much an integral part of society as we are dependent upon them. The many interfaces between us and the billions of animals under our dominion (as well as the environment upon which the welfare of human and non-human animals alike is ultimately dependent) have their separate features: trapping and wildlife management; laboratory animal research; whaling and fishing; veterinary practice; agriculture and farm animal husbandry; horse racing and the ownership of animal companions; the propagation of captive wildlife and their preservation in the wild; the use of animals as companions and for the purposes of vicarious entertainment.

These interfaces are linked by the science of animal welfare which, by virtue of its interdisciplinary nature, includes such disciplines as ethology, veterinary medicine, psychology, physiology, farm animal production technologies; studies of human attitudes towards animals (including cross-cultural anthropology) and the legal protection of animals; humane education, law enforcement, legislation, and ethics of moral philosophy and enlightened self-interest; practical problems such as predator control, euthanasia of unwanted pets and the transportation and slaughter of farm animals; and such issues and questions as animal sentience, sapience, awareness, needs and rights.

Ethics and philosophy have become divorced from science, as values have from facts. Yet ethics and moral philosophy are an integral

*All articles submitted and solicited are subject to refereeing by members of the Manuscript Review Committee (see *Instructions to Authors*).

part of animal welfare science, as are economics, cultural values, perceptions, and social customs. In sum, the scholarly, as distinct from the "objective"*, study of animal welfare embraces all these disciplines and aspects of human-animal relationships. It is a complex and diverse field of inquiry which, through this new annual publication, will gain the international recognition and attention that the subject has long deserved.

*and through the "objectification" of the world, we have achieved considerable power and control over life, yet in the process, have created a multitude of ethical, environmental, social, economic, and other global problems, one major one being the well-being of the animal kingdom.

LIST OF CONTENTS

Part I
Animal Awareness

THE QUESTION OF ANIMAL AWARENESS

Francoise Wemelsfelder

Instituut voor Theoretische Biologie
Groenhovenstraat 5, 2311 BT Leiden
Holland

INTRODUCTION

The problem of animal awareness lies at the interface of science and philosophy. As a starting point for the study of phenomena such as awareness, mind, consciousness, etc., we hardly have any reference other than our *own* human experience and in the context of a non-dualistic ontology this can be justified. In philosophy and psychology it appears to be very difficult to give direct operational definitions of terms such as consciousness, etc. So we might expect this to be even more difficult in the study of animals. A detailed knowledge of animals and their behaviour is necessary in order to be able to say something about their subjective experiences, and to prevent us from excessively projecting human experience on animals.

Descriptive terms dealing with the nature of animal awareness, like intelligence, consciousness, etc., are normative as well (Hodos 1982), and therefore the study of animal awareness has wide-ranging moral implications for our own conduct towards animals (Griffin 1981a; Midgley 1981); some of the reluctance in recognizing the question of animal awareness as legitimate and "scientific" might be explained this way. The question of animal awareness implies the question of the human-animal relationship.

DEFINITIONS

Terms such as awareness, self-awareness, self-consciousness, etc., indicate that there is a gradual scale of awareness rather than distinct "states" of awareness. Each species, and each individual animal within a species, can display different elements of awareness at different times. Roughly speaking, though, the development from lower to higher animals will coincide with an increasing degree of awareness. And, as higher degrees of (self-) awareness are achieved, the more basic forms remain present and functional; they are recapitulated in the development of young individual mammals.

First of all, there is the level of the "un-conscious" or pre-conscious for bodily, e.g. physiological processes, or the maintenance of homeostasis in general. This level is present in all living beings. In conscious life, as opposed to unconscious life, the most basic property seems to be awareness: "a feeling of causal relationship with the external world" (Whitehead, cited by Griffin 1977). This feeling, according to Whitehead, implies discrimination of the quality of the environment (harmful or beneficial) and a sense of location. Down to the lowest forms of life, there are signs of this sort of awareness, be it ever so vague and unspecified. Directly linked to this is the concept of self-hood: "all animals have attained self-hood, since they exist, have a will to survive, and have also needs and interests" (Fox 1983a).

Accepting the idea that perception is basically an "emotional" phenomenon, a "feeling," as Whitehead argues, awareness as defined above is not necessarily equivalent to *mental capacity.* Awareness might be accompanied with the experience of some form of mental images; but by mental capacity is meant the ability to abstract information from external reality in such a way that the dependence of the individual on the environment decreases. "Mind" in this context is more than just the presence of mental images (Gallup 1982, personal communication); it is the capacity to "*use*" these images in a flexible, adaptive way (Griffin 1981b).

Hodos (1982), in a recent review of the concept of intelligence, defines intelligence as a qualitative characterization of an organism's behavioural responses to pressures from the environment, rather than as a "specific intellectual faculty." Being intelligent implies the ability to fulfill purposes, but Hodos' definition stresses the fact that, e.g., a rabbit's purpose might be very different from human purposes.

Along with a growing ability to abstract information about external reality and manipulate the environment instead of being manipulated, a sense of individuality develops as well. Thorpe (1966) refers to self-awareness as individual recognition, of self and others, as a "self." Self-awareness, more than awareness, is the "understanding that I can be the object of another's attentions" (Clark 1981), the ability to see the "self" as another "other" in the environment. While the world in a primary state of self-hood is predominantly subjective, without discrimination between self and other (Fox 1982), the presence of self-awareness in an animal implies its ability to have a relationship with its own body and with its environment, culminating in the experience of an "I" that is not identical with its body nor with its environment. "Self-awareness is the animal's ability to abstract and to form a conceptual framework of its environment, so that it can perceive itself and its actions in relation to the environment" (Wood-Gush 1981).

Self-awareness can become more explicit, and result in still a greater freedom from the environment when self-conscious elements increase; implying the ability to focus attention (Griffin 1981a) or the ability to manipulate ideas (Thorpe 1966). Self-consciousness implies the existence of some sort of introspective ability, the direct experience of the self as self, as a causal agent, not being dominated by sensory brain processes (Thorpe 1966; Sperry 1982). Maybe a clue is that the word "con-scious" comes from the latin verb *scire* meaning "knowing." So "conscious" means "also-knowing": an act performed by a more or less self-conscious being is accompanied by a knowledge of the relativity of the act: its reasons, its purpose, etc. This might be most clearly manifested in the ability to make plans, to act purposefully, or the presence of time-awareness. When consciousness of self increases, then also do the scope of "understanding" and the degree of freedom increase: self-reflectiveness implies the ability to recognize individuality in others due to the fact that other and self are of the same kind (Clark 1981). Moreover it becomes possible to manipulate others (Fox 1982). Capacities like empathy, altruism, intentional deceit, gratitude, etc., are signs of these abilities.

In sum, I propose that any living being has awareness; but an increasing amount of self-awareness entails a splitting of self and other, an ability to discriminate self from not-self, which may be interpreted as the ability to "objectify" (Fox 1982).

In the context of this paragraph it is also important to note that the capacity to suffer could in principle be present well down to the "lower" levels, since awareness is defined as an emotional perception of the quality of the environment to suffering of self-aware beings; yet it indicates that suffering is present not only in self-aware beings.

THE MIND-BODY RELATIONSHIP

The phenomenon of "consciousness," and the existence of an objective "I" has always fascinated man (Lorenz 1963). Is it something that just human beings have, or is the existence of "personality" a universal phenomenon, somehow present in the whole of nature? Different theories have been given to explain the nature of the relationship between "mind" and "body"; within philosophy, it has always been a major topic for study, since it comes so close to the mystery of existence of life itself.

The discussion seems to evolve around two basic perspectives: a dualistic one, in which mind is a separate entity from matter in principle; or a panpsychistic one, which assumes "some sort of psychic element in the ultimate physical particles" (Thorpe 1977).

The dualistic perspective has become very influential since Descartes. In this view, one may regard the mind-body relationship as a two-way causal interaction between mental and physical events (Thorpe 1977). Another form of dualism is the so-called psycho-physical-parellelism theory, in which mental events may be seen as a "side-effect" of physical events (Lorenz 1963).

Since dualism is in essence reductionistic (Thorpe 1977), the question comes up at what point in evolution "mind" came into being and what its adaptive value is in the mechanism of natural selection. Thorpe (1966) stated that "consciousness may have been an evolutionary necessity in that it may have been the only way in which highly complex living organisms could become fully viable." In this way, it would be of great interest to see "whether we can find grounds to think that consciousness is present only above a certain level of neural organization." Thorpe thus seems to follow the widespread intuitive assumption that consciousness is related to complexity of neural organization; and also that it is generated "out of the blue" at a certain point in evolution, through the process of natural selection. Griffin (1981a) also mentions the adaptive value of consciousness for complex animals, in order to cope with changing situations. He goes on, however, arguing that "a sufficiently fertile imagination can almost always find a plausible adaptive advantage for any observed trait," and therefore the argument for the adaptive value of consciousness is not very weighty in the consideration of its existence. Humphrey (1982) expresses his doubt of complexity as a condition for consciousness by saying that our animal ancestors "were no doubt percipient, intelligent, complexily motivated creatures, whose internal control mechanisms were in many respects the equals of our own. But it is to say that they had no way of looking in upon the mechanism. They had clever brains, but blank minds." He proposes social complexity as a reason for the sudden appearance of consciousness.

Arguments against dualistic perspectives are that one can speculate about possible parameters for the generation of consciousness, but these remain scientifically unverifiable, and ultimately the existence of life itself becomes an unexplainable event in a dualistic framework.

"Generally, in the building of a scientifically 'sound' theory, we want the newly apparent property to be explicable in terms of the old,...to be the sum of whatever composes it...So the awareness of a complex organism ought, we feel, to be a similar resultant, and either atoms are already conscious, or else consciousness is only a misleading label for neural impulse'' (Nagel, cited by Clarke 1981). ''There must be something positive limiting chance, and something more than mere matter in matter, or Darwinism fails to explain life'' (Hartshorne, cited by Birch 1974). Others, however, reject the idea of ''panpsychism'' as ''cheap'' and ''a radical simplification'' (Popper 1974), or because it is not possible to confirm this idea scientifically, and that there is no visible evidence that lower life forms are conscious, as are humans and some higher animals (Thorpe 1977).

There is, however, a third perspective possible. It is a concept in some ways resembling panpsychism, yet it is also fundamentally different. Whitehead has developed a theory in which events are at the same time both mental and physical. Thorpe (1977) states that Whitehead is a panpsychist, yet this does not seem the case to me. The idea that all ''life-events'' are physical and mental *by nature*, does not imply that these events are conscious of this, as panpsychism implies. Nor does the idea that perception and physical energy are emotional in nature, imply that this emotionality is consciously experienced at the lower levels.

A theory which defined the nature of life processes as both physical and mental, in a meaningful interaction, provides a basis for a gradually evolving continuum of mental capacity. The fact that we accept the statement ''human beings are conscious'' more or less as an axiom (Lorenz 1980), forces us to accept that we most probably share this quality at least *rudimentarily* with most life forms (Fox 1976; Griffin 1981a; Rollin 1981; Lorenz 1980).

To account for the evolution of a rudimentary form of perception of causal relationships, to a conscious experience of self is not easy, and still requires the explanation of ''leaps,'' for example between the occurence of mental images and the use of a real mind, as defined above.

The results of the research on split brains and the nature of consciousness by Nobel-prize winner Roger Sperry (1982) point in the direction of an explanatory concept known as ''the emergent principle.'' It implies that interaction between parts creates a ''whole'' that has intrinsic qualities of its own which none of the parts possess. In Whitehead's framework, this element of ''the whole being more than the sum of the parts'' is equivalent to the subjective, ''mental'' part of events. ''The key development is a switch...to a new causal or interactionist interpretation that ascribes to the inner experience an integral causal control role in brain function and behaviour...The whole, besides being 'different from, and greater than the sum of the parts,'... also causally determines the fates of the parts, without interfering with the physical or chemical laws of subentities at their own level.

The events of inner experience as emergent properties of brain processes, become themselves explanatory causal constructs in their own right." (Sperry 1982).

These results are derived from research on human beings, and therefore mainly apply to them. A much wider range of application of the main principles is clearly indicated, however; Sperry himself states that the acceptance of the revised causal view has important implications for scientific views of man and nature. Also he says that his results indicate features about the nature of consciousness and its fundamental relation to "brain processing." Unless we suppose that the general concept of animal consciousness is completely different from human consciousness, which is extremely unlikely (Fox 1976; Midgley 1978; Griffin 1981a), it is only reasonable to apply general principles about "the nature of consciousness" to animals as well, and in a Whiteheadian framework to all evolutionary events in general.

If this is the case, then however simple the nervous mechanism might be, there will always be generated "a whole," some sort of inner experience.

Complexity of nervous structure probably correlates to complexity of inner experience (Fox 1976). The more complex the interaction between parts, which then in turn can serve as a new part, of a new emergent quality, a new "whole." But it would be a mistake to set up a simple hierarchy of values, attributed to different sorts of complexity (Hodos 1982). Rather, all life forms constitute "an integrated, interdependent unified field of being, not a ladder leading to some ultimate goal of perfection." (Fox personal communication 1982).

What an emergent "whole" seems to express is "the being-ness" of a certain animal, e.g., "the dogness" that comes out of the specific neural organization of a dog. This beingness implies consciousness on its own level, on its dog-, or fish-, or whale-level. Each "beingness" has its own, unique qualities to contribute to the overall ecosystem and possesses unique modes of perception and awareness, suitable for the needs of the animal (Hodos 1982).

In conclusion, we can say that man is not alone on earth in his awareness of life around him; all life forms are conscious in their own, unique way, and the capacity to individualize and become self-aware gradually emerges from the lowest levels of perception.

Philosophically speaking, the possibility for real sensitivity and awareness in the animal kingdom is given. Now we must see what the biological study of awareness leads to in the framework of a nondualistic philosophy.

In the biological study of awareness, the main indicator for "beingness" would be behaviour, since it represents that aspect of an animal in which all partial aspects, like physiological and hormonal processes, are integrated; it also includes the subjective, individual evaluation of all these partial aspects. Behaviour, being itself an emergent property, is the nearest indicator of the animal's emergent individual subjectivity and quality of being. In fact, one could say that behaviour is the overt, outward manifestation of inner experience, both being on the same level of emergence.

An animal relates to its environment through its behaviour. It expresses its inner drives, abilities, and experiences in the way it deals with different environmental influences. We, as "human animals," can evaluate different kinds of behaviour by observation and experiments, and try to classify the quality of beingness as "aware," "self-aware," "intelligent," etc. The behavioural data available for this will now be discussed.

THE ANIMAL AND ITS ENVIRONMENT

The great "oneness" between animal and environment, the complete adaptation which makes animals fit right into their specific "niche," has caused some scientists to presume that animals are automata, blindly ruled by environmental circumstances. The other, opposite, way of looking at it is that animals are so perfectly aware of their environment and at one with it, that an almost transcendent unity arises. In this view the essence of animal life lies largely in its relation to the surrounding world, and this notion leads "phenomenological" scientists to say that the subjectivity of an animal lies as it were in its "Umwelt" and a *qualitative* study of the way an animal "meets" its environment is the basis for understanding the animal's experiential world, as well as its ecological function (Kortlandt 1954).

This qualitative beingness of an animal is called its *nature*, or "*telos*" (Midgley 1978; Rollin 1981), implying the unique expression of life that a species represents, and the specificity of needs and purposes of each different species.

D.R. Griffin should receive the credit for having opened the door again to serious scientific investigation into animal awareness with his book *The Question of Animal Awareness* (1981a). With respect to animal learning, one of the most basic properties of animal life, he suggests that the principle of parsimony might be best served by accepting some sort of awareness related to animal learning. Trying to stick to the behaviourist standpoint that animals are black boxes leads to "complex circumlocutions and confusing euphemisms," which are "far less parsimonious than frankly calling a spade a spade and a thought a thought."

The ability to learn is one of the most basic properties of animal life. In his review on animal intelligence, Hodos (1982) states that habituation "appears to be a universal phenomenon in animal organisms, including protozoans." Also "classical-and operant conditioning have been demonstrated...in those metazoans that possess a central nervous system with axial symmetry." This includes platyhelminthes (e.g., planarians), annelids, arthropods and molluscs. Delayed response as a more complex behaviour has been reported in arthropods and molluscs, and molluscs are also capable of reversal learning, so Hodos reports.

A well-known anecdote that Buytendijk reports is that an octopus is able to distinguish between "touching" and "being touched," which might even indicate the presence of self-awareness: "A good example of a lower animal with highly developed interactions with its environment is the octopus, which has a highly differentiated set of behaviour, much more so than some vertebrates...One could attribute a relatively clear form of consciousness to an octopus...The fact that an octopus has so-called pupil-reactions e.g. in adverse situations, an indication of emotional life in mammals, could imply a high degree of development" (Buytendijk 1963).

Entomologist V.B. Wiggelsworth in a recent article argued that insects might experience visceral pain, as well as pain caused by heat and electric shock (Rollin 1981). From the existing literature it can be argued that the experience of pain as such is not possible without the presence of some sort of purely subjective, inner experience, since the adversity of any stimulus is essentially something which is experienced subjectively.

Given the fact that awareness seems to exist from the "lowest" level of animal life onward, it develops and becomes more complex along with the development of neural complexity, as was stated earlier. But do animals come near to any kind of "higher" awareness at all, any kind of the faculties we consider "intelligent" and self-aware in humans? More than anything else, introspection and the use of symbols are regarded as specific human characteristics, which set man apart from all other living beings (Jeuken 1975).

GENERAL INTELLIGENT BEHAVIOUR

The ability to make use of symbols is related to a number of other abilities: to use language, to use concepts, to have time-awareness, and to respond adequately to novelty, amongst others. It implies a capacity to abstract from present reality, and in that respect is directly linked to introspection, which is the capacity to regard the self in an abstract, "symbolic" way. Many authors connect introspection with social communication (Humphrey 1978; Midgley 1978; Griffin 1981a;

Thorpe 1966), or with intention-behaviour and imitation (Rollin 1981; Midgley 1978). These are mostly the topics dealt with by authors who discuss animal awareness. They support their point of view with evidence coming from either the little amount of systematic research being done in this field, or from anecdotes of "natural," "spontaneous" behaviour. A few relevant examples of this evidence will be given shortly.

Griffin (1981a) states that "Black, McMullan, Robinson, and others have distinguished animal communication systems from human language on the ground that the former are rigid responses to external or internal stimuli, which...be definitely specified, whereas human language is spontaneous, creative and unpredictable." The animal's ability to communicate may be less rigid, however, since studies of animal behaviour have shown that animals are also capable of spontaneous, creative and unpredictable behaviour. For example, Markowitz (1982), in his book on behavioural enrichment in zoos, reports the highly unique, creative, unpredictable way in which zoo animals would invent solutions and play games. A young elephant, for instance, instead of touching the right panel to set off an electrically regulated reward, would always save water in his trunk, no matter how long before the experimental session the trough was emptied, and smear the water between the response panels, thereby electrically shorting them, so that every response would pay off. (The same elephant walked over to the only arrogant, boasting person in a group of students and stepped deliberately on this person's foot). This story, in which the animal actually manipulates the research project and the researcher, instead of the other way around, can hardly be interpreted otherwise than as a falsification of the argument presented by the three researchers in Griffin's book. It gives evidence of the presence of time-awareness ("I will use this water *later*"), intentionality, conceptual thinking and creativity in handling a completely new situation, and its behaviour therefore is worthy to be labelled consciously self-aware.

All of this also holds for a story that Rollin (1981) reports of a police dog who was trained to hold suspects by the arm unharmed until the officer arrived. When they ran into a robbery being performed by two men, the men broke away and took off in different directions, assuming the dog could not pursue both. The dog chased one of them, disabled his leg, left him, ran after the other and held this man unharmed by his arm, in this way having caught both men, although he never had been trained to attack the leg. Like Fox (1982), Mugford (1981) concludes that the ability to manipulate matters in order to fulfill a need, gives evidence of self-awareness. Many dog owners may be able to give examples of dogs who manipulate their owners. Dolphins, apes (Midgley 1978), wolves (Fox 1974), etc., are able to save wounded fellows and humans, use and invent tools, and deceive prey in order to catch it. Both Markowitz and Mugford stress the fact that in these situations the animal is in control, rather than the experimenter, and that by humbling himself in this way, the observer might "investigate ways in which animals derive unique solutions, rather than simply measuring their activities in a narrow response largely dictated by the experimenter." (Markowitz 1982). However, there are also *experiments* that indicate some sort of awareness in different animals. Dawkins (1980) describes well-known experiments with pigeons and rats. Beninger and his co-workers trained rats to indicate what behaviour they were performing at the moment a buzzer was sounding. They tried to find a simpler hypothesis than that the rats were actually aware of what they were doing, but failed to do so. This experiment strongly suggests even a kind of conscious awareness in rats. Hernstein and Loveland, and Siegel and Honig, proved by showing numerous slides to pigeons that they are capable of forming what could be described as abstract concepts of almost anything, like water, trees, human beings, etc.; Kohler furthermore found by doing ingenious, well-controlled tests that pigeons can count, or as he put it, "think unnamed numbers," and in doing this, really grasp the concept of numbers, rather than being "Clever Hanses." (Clever Hans was a horse who could do many a mathematical calculation, but later it was discovered that he reacted to subtle indications of his owner, instead of calculating.)

It seems that this evidence, experimental and anecdotal, shows that some animals are fully capable of abstraction and that they can think symbolically in order to express themselves and control their world. What about the "highest" form of symbolic communication, namely language?

LANGUAGE

There is no consensus about the real nature of language, let alone the difference between man and animals in this respect. Chomsky (cited by Griffin 1981a), argues that "the unboundness of human speech, as an expression of limitless thought, is an entirely different matter (from animal communication), because of the freedom from stimulus control and the appropriateness to new situations." Griffin comments that animal communication is not that rigid at all, nor is human language endless in its scope. Midgley (1978) considers speech as a further development of "creative, expressive, communicative power," and nothing all by itself. Fox (1976) relates speech to the controlling and predicting function of the rational mind, which does not diminish the consciousness and deep emotional experiences that the intuitive mind can have, without speaking a word. Animals can very well have such an intuitive kind of mentality. In this line, Rollin (1981) argues, while discussing the "private language argument" developed by Wittgenstein, that animals might have to rely far more on direct experience for learning than on words, or that they might express their universal statements (all strangers are dangerous) by their behaviour instead of words, but that this does not imply that animals are not rational beings; rational being defined as the ability to do the right thing at a certain moment, choosing between different possibilities (Rollin 1981; Midgley 1978). In any case, the fact that the possession of a communication system is a widespread property rather than a specific human trait, might be demonstrated by the ability of the chimpanzees trained by the Gardners (Griffin 1981a) to express themselves in a language-like way with gestures, and acquire the "vocabulary" of a young human child.

Also, dolphins have been shown to be able to communicate certain instructions to a mate purely by sound, while they could not see each other (Fichtelius and Sjölander 1972).

Monkeys are known to have different warning calls for predators in the air or on the ground (Seyfarth 1982). The explicit use of variation in sound for communication, with which apparently detailed and precise information can be passed on, comes very close to what we call "language."

SOCIAL ORGANIZATION

Rather than attributing self-awareness only to language-using species, many authors discuss the likelihood, and the need, for self-awareness in all *socially organized species*. Social animals, dependent on each other for survival, must understand the other animals and their mental state in order to act adequately (Humphrey 1978); or must be able to recognize other individuals in relation to themselves in order to maintain a hierarchy, as in the case of domestic pigs, cattle and chickens (Bryant 1972), or to live in families or clans (Thorpe 1966). Fox (1974) describes altruistic behaviour in wolf clans: wolves that go hunting bring back food for the cubs and the "babysitters" that remained behind.

In the growing up of young animals, play and imitation are of great importance. The great ability of young (and older) animals to play indicates their need for the capacity to be aware of self and others, the need to be able to react to new situations and make decisions; play facilitates the development of these capacities. But apart from the functional meaning of play, it implies that animals are spontaneous, creative and sentient beings, individuals who are fully able to enjoy themselves.

While it is sometimes suggested that it is a proof of an animal's "dumbness" that it imitates a researcher, instead of "consciously" performing acts, authors like Thorpe, Midgley and Fox refer to play and imitation as crucial for healthy development in the more complex social animals, and as a clear indication of the animal's ability to engage in creative, highly communicative action. The "teaching" of the art of survival by parents to their offspring could even be seen as a beginning of culture (Fox 1976). Bonner (1980) devotes a whole book to "culture" in animal species.

Roughly speaking, the presence of "animal awareness" in its many forms has been discussed by going into the phenomena of learning behaviour, general intelligent behaviour, communicative behaviour and social behaviour.

Now that the question "can animals think?" has been discussed, an equal amount could be written on the question "can animals feel?" However, I will not attempt it, since many of the same principles that apply to awareness, apply to the existence of emotions, and the two are intimately, perhaps inseparably, linked together in animal behaviour.

ANIMAL FEELINGS

As a fact of life, feelings must be rudimentarily present in all life forms, as Whitehead philosophically indicated. Basic emotions like fear, aggression, frustration, and satisfaction are directly related to internal motivational states (Wiepkema 1982) and are essential for the survival of the animal (Dawkins 1977; Murphy 1978; van Putten 1981). For instance, fear in the predator-prey relationship is very essential. Considerable research on fear in the domestic chicken has been done by researchers like Hughes and Murphy (Murphy 1978).* The fact that these "instincts" have a biological function, and in that respect might be predictable, does not in the least imply the absence of an actual emotional experience (Clark 1981; Dawkins 1977; van Rooyen 1981). As the selfhood of animals develops into greater degrees of self-awareness it will be accompanied by a greater capacity for individual, conscious emotion. This is especially evident in social animals, who often form life-long bonds with mates or clans (Fox 1976). Well-known examples are swans, geese and ducks who choose a partner for the rest of their lives. Lorenz (1980) describes the signs of grief shown by a goose

---

*See also *Fear in Animals and Man*, 1979. W. Sluckin (ed). New York: Van Nostrand Reinhold,—Ed.

when it looses its mate; for instance its eyes become dull, its muscles weaken and the goose lets its head hang down, just as people do, so Lorenz comments. He states that higher mammals and birds have emotional experiences completely similar to ours, representative of the basic structure of all experiences for man and animal alike (Lorenz 1980; see also Midgley 1978). Self-awareness of the emotional state is shown by the chimpanzee Lucy, who possessed learned gesture-language; during a session, when her foster mother went away, she ran to a window and signed to herself: "cry me, me cry" (Midgley 1978). She was also able to appreciate jokes, and imitate them for her own amusement.

Emotions can also lead to empathetic (altruistic) action, such as cases where dogs save little children, and dolphins support a sick or injured companion. Emotions must also underly the "psychic" tracking of dogs who travel hundreds of miles to find their owners who moved to a place, unknown (!) before the dog's arrival (Fox 1976). Because of the similarity in emotional make-up, animals have many of the same psychological illnesses and abnormalities as humans, e.g. anorexia and depression, which in higher animals can occur as a result of sudden environmental changes, such as captivity and isolation from peers, mate or parent (Fox 1971). Carter (1982), for example, presents evidence which indicates strongly that many causes of death for dolphins in captivity are psycho-physiological, the shock of captivity being the cause for a loss of resistance to disease. Sometimes psychoneurotic illness can be the result of captivity or loss of a mate. This is also the basis for the very extensive research that is being done on animals in laboratories, using them as models for human disorders. Research to find new drugs to relieve anxiety is often done on mice and rats (Goodman and Gilman 1975; McKegney 1982). The experiments of Suomi and Harlow on the development of depression as a result of maternal deprivation are also well known. They developed "a monkey model of human anaclictic depression, since...the resulting behaviours are seemingly identical for monkey and human infants alike" (Midgley 1981). Because of this correspondence in structure and behaviour Midgley is right, I think, when she criticizes such experiments from an ethical point of view.

Midgley (1978) comments that "to be disposed to make the gestures, you must also be capable of the emotions in order for them to be convincing and truly reciprocal;" "behaviour is only possible for a creature with an inward dimension, with its own real perception of the world." (Clark 1981). However, the mind is a private thing, as so many scientists comment (Griffin 1981a), for humans and animals alike; and so the gap remains, however much research and interpretation we are prepared to do. At least humans can speak and explain their thoughts and feelings. But animals cannot; or can they?

Lorenz (1963, 1980) states that the similarity of experience, the direct comparability of one's own experience with that of others is beyond proof, in that it is so evident that we cannot *not* believe it. This extends at least to higher vertebrates. Karl Buhler, according to Lorenz, refers to this as "*du-evidenz,*" a necessary axiom of life. It is not up to science to establish the framework of communication and recognition of behaviour, or have "heady metaphysical doubt" about the similarity of experience of man and man, and man and animal, since science itself depends on this mutual understanding (Clark 1981). He goes on to say that "we do not see merely material motions (of an animal) but rather the embodiment of character and feeling in a material mode." To make use of the so-called analogy-postulate to assume animal awareness (Sambraus 1981) might not be direct enough. The fact that we really *do* see the embodiment of character and feelings in behaviour (Clark 1981; Midgley 1978; Fox 1983b) makes it not only justified to describe "material entities in mentalistic terms" (Clark 1981) but we have no right to *withhold* those terms to describe animal behaviour (Rollin 1982, personal communication). "Stones cannot be bored, or cross, or joyful, but dogs and pigs and cattle can" (Clark 1981).

In an overall perspective, we might say that animals are alive, and present in their beingness, for anyone who wants to see and meet them on their own ground. What their minds, or inner experiences are like, is largely expressed in their behaviour in intimate interaction with the environment, including other individuals. Olfactory and auditory senses might play as great a role in this interaction as the highly valued visual senses (Fox 1976). Although it seems to bother many scientists that many of the abilities ascribed to animals are also attributable to machines, the nature of the machine is given to it by man, and the parts are equally as independent or durable as the whole; when an animal dies, however, the whole body dies, which again shows the causality of the whole, and the fundamental selfhood of a whole organism (Rollin 1981).

We, as human beings, share different traits with different species (Midgley 1978) and are especially close to the more complex social animals such as dogs, elephants, dolphins, and apes, in that those seem to have a highly developed self-awareness and even self-reflectiveness. Besides, we are able to communicate with them, to a great extent, as one individual to another.

Human beings belong to the "*Umwelt*" of an animal, just as animals belong to ours. It is in the *meeting* of individual and *Umwelt*, of man and animal, that mutual understanding and appreciation grows (Kortlandt 1954). There is no separation between our position as observer and as partner in the relationship and in this context it can be seen how our understanding of animals has a direct moral impact on our actions.

The fact that it is justifiable to describe animal behaviour in empathetic terms does not imply at all that "scientific" inquiry in the form of systematic observation would not be necessary and useful. It is important in order to discover the nature of different animal species, and systematically investigate different assumptions about their nature, needs, and interests.

The most instructive and direct way to learn about animals is by observing their *spontaneous* behaviour under conditions where they have total freedom to express themselves to their fullest potential (Midgley 1978; Markowitz 1982). "Despite the difficulties, field work with gorillas, chimpanzees, orangutans, and wolves demonstrates that the most realistic observations and assessments on wild animals are those made in the natural environment" (Carter 1982). For other animals, for example dogs and cats, a man-made environment can provide an adequate situation in which a personal bond between observer and animal might well be a very valuable way of testing and understanding an animal (Mugford 1981; Fox 1983b).

Working in the experimental environment of a laboratory the danger is great that the knowledge which is produced "is hardly a wholesome source of learning, since it is based on abnormally conditioned animals" (Carter 1982). The most important thing is to ask the *right* question, so that the animal can show us its abilities. A negative answer to a test, like Gallup's mirror-tests, might be our fault: we did not ask the correct question for that particular species (Rees, Wolfle 1982, personal communication).

The capacities of an animal to feel and be aware are not static states by themselves, but abilities that are constantly expressed and developed in interaction among animal, man and environment.

CONSEQUENCES FOR THE FIELD OF ANIMAL WELFARE

A being who is aware of his environment, and can react emotionally to external situations, is also able to suffer. Every level of "beingness" has its own purpose and needs, and its own qualitative link with its environment; the thwarting of those needs matters to an animal, and most animals will struggle to survive if in danger. The whole notion of the nature, or telos, of an animal implies that it will suffer if a certain level of "fulfillment" of its behavioural possibilities is not reached. In relation to animals in present intensive production systems, Humphrey (1981) points out the importance of realizing that domestic animals have become "dull" and unresponsive not because they are dumb and stupid but because we have made them that way by depriving them of stimuli which would enable them to develop a proper sense of selfhood.

The suggestion that domestic animals do not miss what they do not know is rejected because the concept of animal awareness implies that animals actually *experience* suffering in some conscious way. The absence of human-like self-consciousness might even increase the intensity of animal suffering: most animals cannot foresee whether their situation will improve or not, nor realize other factors which make their suffering relative. Because of this lack of knowledge, all that may exist for them is a feeling of suffering.

An animal, whether a "lower" or a "higher" one, is a qualitative, sentient being. To affect its environment is to affect the quality of its existence, and its individual well-being.

Current intensive production systems have affected what used to be the natural environment of farm animals tremendously. The demand for efficiency and production more and more became the guiding factor in designing and creating living environments for the animals. As a result, environmental diversity has been reduced to its absolute minimum. The reaction of animals, dependent on the environment as they are for their development and health, to this deprivation, will be detailed later in Section IV of this book (*Animal Management*, Wemelsfelder).

REFERENCES

Birch, C. 1974. Chance, necessity and purpose. In: Ayala, F.J. and Dobzhansky, T. eds. *Studies in the philosophy of biology*. Berkeley:University of California Press.

Bonner, J.T. 1980. *The evolution of culture in animals*. Princeton, New Jersey: Princeton University Press.

Bryant, M.J. 1972. The social environment: behaviour and stress in housed livestock. *Vet.Rec.* 90(13):351-9.

Buyjtendijk, F.J. 1963. *Over de pijn*. 5e ed. Utrecht:Aula.

Carter, N. 1982. Effect of psycho-physiological stress on captive dolphins. *Int.J. Stud.Anim.Prob.* 3(3):193-8.

Clark, S.R.L. 1981. Awareness and self-awareness. In: Wood-Gush, D.G.M., Dawkins, M. and Ewbank, R., eds. *Self-awareness in domesticated animals*. Hertfordshire: UFAW.

Dawkins, M.S. 1977. Do hens suffer in battery cages? Environmental preferences and welfare. *Animal Beh.* 25:1034-46.

Dawkins, M.S. 1980. *Animal suffering. The science of animal welfare*. London, New York:Chapman and Hall.

Fichtelius, K.E. and Sjölander, S. 1972. *Smarter than man? Intelligence in whales, dolphins and humans*. New York: Pantheon Books.

Fox, M.W. 1971. Psychopathology in man and lower animals. *J.A.V.M.A.* 159(1):66-77.

Fox, M.W. 1974. *Concepts in ethology*. Minneapolis:University of Minnesota Press.

Fox, M.W. 1976. *Between animal and man*. New York:Coward, McCann and Geoghegan, Inc.

Fox, M.W. 1982. Are most animals "mindless automatons"?: A reply to Gordon G. Gallup, Jr. *Amer.J.Primatol.* 3:341-3.

Fox, M.W. 1983a. *Farm animals: Husbandry, behaviour and veterinary care: Viewpoints of a critic*. Baltimore: University Park Press.

Fox, M.W. 1983b. Scientific objectivity and the subjective world. In:Rowan, A., ed. *Animal awareness—human perceptions: implications for animal welfare*. Albany, New York:In press. State University of New York.

Goodman, L.S. and Gilman, A. 1975. *The pharmacological basis of therapeutics*. New York:McMillan and Co., Inc.

Griffin, D.R. 1977. Whitehead's philosophy and some general notions of physics and biology. In Cobb. J.B. and Griffin, D.R., eds. *Mind in nature*. Washington, D.C.: University Press of America.

Griffin, D.R. 1981a. *The question of animal awareness*. 2nd. ed. New York:The Rockefeller University Press.

Griffin, D.R. 1981b. The problem of distinguishing awareness from responsiveness. In: Wood-Gush, D.G.M., Dawkins, M., and Ewbank, R., eds. *Self-awareness in domesticated animals*. Hertfordshire:UFAW.

Hodos, W. 1982. Some perspectives on the evolution of intelligence and the brain. In: Griffin, D.R., ed. *Animal mind—human mind*. Berlin, New York:Springer-Verlag.

Humphrey, N. 1978. Nature's psychologist. *New Scientist* 78:900-03.

Humphrey, N. 1981. In:Wood-Gush, D.G.M., Dawkins, M. and Ewbank, R., eds. *Self-awareness in domesticated animals*. Hertfordshire: UFAW, general discussion, pp. 10,50.

Humphrey, N. 1982. Consciousness: a just so story. *New Scientist* 19 August:474-7.

Jeuken, M. 1975. Het dier in het menselijk milieu. *Tijdschr. Diergeneesk.* 100 (13): 692-6.

Kortlandt, A. 1954. Cosmologie der dieren. *Vakbl. voor Biol.* 34(1):1-14.

Lorenz, K. 1963. Haben Tiere ein subjektives Erleben? In: Lorenz, K. *Gesammelte abhandlungen II:uber tierischer und menschlicher*. München:Verhalten, Piper and Co.

Lorenz, K. 1980. Die technomorphe Behandlung von Tieren. *Sonderdruck nr. 2. Arbeitsgemeinschaft* Deutscher Tierschutz eV.

Markowitz, H. 1982. *Behavioural enrichment in the zoo.* New York, London:Van Nostrand Reinhold Co.

McKegney, F.P. 1982. Psychoneuro-immunology. What lies ahead. *Drug Therapy.* August:25-35.

Midgley, M. 1978. *Beast and man.* New York:New American Library.

Midgley, M. 1981. Why knowledge matters. In:Sperlinger, D., ed. *Animals in research.* New York:John Wiley and Sons.

Mugford, R.A. 1981. The social skills of dogs as an indicator of animal awareness. In: Wood-Gush, D.G.M., Dawkins, M. and Ewbank, R., eds. *Self-awareness in domesticated animals.* Hertfordshire:UFAW.

Murphy, L.B. 1978. The practical problems of recognizing and measuring fear and exploration behaviour in the domestic fowl. *Anim.Behav.* 26:422-31.

Popper, K.R. 1974. Scientific reduction and the essential incompleteness of all science. In:Ayala, F.J. and Dobzhansky, T. eds. *Study in the philosophy of biology.* Berkeley:University of California Press.

Putten, G. van. 1981. Het meten van welzijn bij landbouwhuisdieren. *Tijdschr. Diergeneesk.* 106(3):106-18.

Rollin, B.E. 1981. *Animal rights and human morality.* New York: Prometheus Books.

Rooyen, J. van. 1981. Are feelings adaptations? The basis of modern applied animal ethology. *Appl. Anim. Ethol.* 7:187-9.

Sambraus, H.H. 1981. Beurteilung von Verhaltens-anomalien aus ethologischer Sicht. *2 GFT-Seminar fur angewandte Nutztierethologie Bayerische Landesanstalt fur Tierzucht,* Grub:1-9.

Seyfarth, R.M. 1982. Communication as evidence of thinking. State of the art report. In:Griffin, D.R., ed. *Animal mind—human mind.* Berlin, New York:Dahlem Konferenzen. Springer-Verlag.

Sperry, R. 1982. Some effect of disconnecting the cerebral hemispheres. *Science* 217: 1223-6.

Thorpe, W.H. 1966. Ethology and consciousness. In:Eccles, J.C., ed. *Brain and conscious experience.* Berlin:Springer-Verlag.

Thorpe, W.H. 1977. The frontiers of biology. Does process thought help? In: Cobb, J.B. and Griffin, D.R., eds. *Mind in nature.* Washington, D.C.: University Press of America.

Wiepkema, P.R. 1982. On the identity and significance of disturbed behavior in vertebrates. In: Bessei, W., ed. *Disturbed behavior in farm animals.* Höhenheimer Arbeitz Heft 121. Eugen Ulmer Verlag, Stuttgart.

Wood-Gush, D.G.M. 1981. In: Wood-Gush, D.G.M., Dawkins, M., Ewbank, R., eds. *Self-awareness in domesticated animals,* General discussion. Hertfordshire: UFAW.

Part II
Human/Animal Relationships

THE ORIGINS OF EMPATHY AND ALTRUISM

Carolyn Zahn-Waxler, Barbara Hollenbeck and Marian Radke-Yarrow

National Institute of Mental Health
Bethesda, MD 20205

Empathy and altruism are most commonly thought of as forms of compassion that human beings express toward one another. However, emotions and behaviors reflecting apparent concern for others occur within other species and across species as well. Although not without controversy, ethologists and sociobiologists (e.g., Wilson 1975) have identified many behaviors in other animals and insects that may be viewed as prosocial or altruistic (e.g., cooperative efforts of bees, warning calls of many species, rescue behaviors of whales, certain acts of mammalian caregivers toward their young, etc.). There are fewer signs of altruism across species. Some animals can be trained to protect, defend and help others (usually humans) in distress. Animal owners sometimes indicate that their pets show emotional concern for others. In observing parent-child interaction in the home we have seen emotionally distressed pets hovering over persons feigning distress in situations where we are measuring the *child's* capacity for empathy. The recent spate of research on animal facilitated therapy attests to the capacity of animals to provide comfort to persons suffering from a variety of physical and emotional problems.

Altruism across species is probably most commonly seen, however, in human behavior toward other animals. Humans are known to help, comfort, share with, protect and defend animals. There have even been reports of loss of human life, for example, in the process of rescuing animals. There is also enormous variation among humans in their sensitivity to their own animals, their commitment to principles of humane treatment, (Miller 1983) and their concern for preservation of wildlife. It is difficult to account for these individual differences in human beings' capacities for compassionate versus aggressive, exploitative attitudes and behaviors toward others, for the origins are multiple and complex.

In a review of the altruism literature, Burleson (in press) concluded that comforting activity by humans is most likely to occur or occurs more sensitively when the distressed, needy other (a) has a close, caring relationship with the comforter, (b) shows salient signs of distress, and (c) is perceived by the comforter as similar to himself or herself. In order to facilitate altruism then, it would be important, to identify both the attributes we have in common with others (animal as well as human) and the factors that promote caring relationships. The earlier in development the emotional ties are established, presumably the more deeply engrained will be the compassion. The purpose of this chapter is to explore these processes in greater detail.

We will describe theories and research that try to explain the development, especially in children, of sensitivity to the needs of others. Are children born with empathy? Is it instinctive or learned? What kinds of changes do humane feelings and behaviors undergo as children develop? How do the environments in which children are reared determine whether they will be more or less likely to show concern and to assume responsibility for the welfare of others? We have examined these issues in a series of studies of (a) the early origins of emotional concern (empathy) and (b) the translation of concerned *feelings* into altruistic behaviors such as helping, sharing, and comforting. Because of an interest in the development of *generalized* altruism, we have studied children's prosocial orientations toward humans and animals, in many settings and over long intervals of time. We will consider the implications of theories and research findings for humane attitudes and treatment.

Empathy refers to the capacity to feel what another is feeling. Examples include the sadness felt when tragedy strikes a friend or the pleasure vicariously experienced in relation to another's joy. It is, then, the sharing of an emotional experience. While it is not restricted to the contagion of any particular emotion, the term most commonly does refer to the emotional concern aroused by the suffering of another living being. This is where our research interest has centered—on the development of emotions and behaviors reflecting concern for the welfare of others. Empathy has many functions. It is viewed by some as essential to all social interactions and relationships because it informs us about the inner world of the other person (Meade 1934). It has been suggested that empathy is critical to the process of insight, for one sees oneself through the eyes of the other via empathy (Dymond 1945). In some theories of moral development (e.g., Hogan 1973) empathy is a necessary component of mature, moral functioning. Empathy may be a fundamental motivator in eliciting altruistic and prosocial behaviors and inhibiting aggressive ones (Hoffman 1976; Feshbach and Feshbach, in press). And empathy is viewed as a critical condition of effective therapeutic intervention in psychotherapy (Rogers 1957) and psychoanalysis (Olinick 1980).

Empathy is hypothesized to have both a cognitive and affective component, i.e., (a) the emotional experiencing or sensing of the other's experience and (b) the intellectual understanding or interpretation of what that experience means (Hoffman 1976). In very young children and in animals as well, where symbolic capacities are limited, we would expect the emotional component of empathy to predominate. In theory, both the cognitive and emotional aspects of empathy should enhance the likelihood of caring for another in need and hence of assuring humane treatment. And with increases in intellectual abilities and competencies throughout childhood, compassionate behavior, too, should increase. However, this is not always the case. Another person's distress may be so frightening or painful when experienced empathically, that it may turn the viewer away from the victim's plight. Intense emotional involvement and preoccupation with another's problems may enmesh one in that distress so completely that it interferes with appropriate emotional concern and provision of constructive help. Further, we may mistakenly project our own emotions onto another with whom we think we are empathizing. Finally, knowledge of another's needs, emotions, and desires may be used to manipulate or control another person, to prey on their vulnerabilities, or to intellectualize, and hence deny, the experience.

Prosocial behaviors, acts that benefit another in need (e.g., help, sharing, cooperation, comfort, protection, rescue, and defense) also represent complex and diverse processes. They may or may not be the behavioral counterparts to feelings of concern. Helping can be an intrusive and unwanted act of domination, defense of a victim often contains elements of aggression and anger, sharing may be done with expectations of reciprocity, comforting may be motivated by guilt or righteous indignation, cooperation may be in the services of intent ultimately to exploit a partner. These complexities suggest (a) that there may be optimal levels of expression of concerned feelings and behaviors, and (b) that some types of prosocial behavior are more likely than others to reflect altruism or generalized humane behavior. It is important to try to distinguish those emotions and behaviors that reflect genuine concern, because this attribute is particularly important in assuring humane treatment.

THEORIES OF THE DEVELOPMENT OF EMPATHY AND ALTRUISM

There are four major theories that have been used to explain the development of altruism. They variously emphasize the importance of (1) guilt and conscience, (2) cognitive development, (3) instinct, and (4) learning and environmental processes, to explain the origins and maintenance of prosocial behavior.

PSYCHOANALYTIC THEORY

In psychoanalytic theory, the concept of identification has been used to explain how the values and mores of society become internalized, and hence why children become prosocial. The child is believed to become altruistic, to share and cooperate, either because of guilt resulting from moral transgressions or through the internalization of ego ideals (i.e., positively valued behaviors in others). The concept of pathological altruism also derives from psychoanalytic theory. The emphasis is on unconscious, inner forces that drive the behaviors. This approach has produced relatively few studies, but it seems reasonable to assume that prosocial behaviors (e.g., help sharing and comfort) for some persons and on some occasions result from feelings of guilt or an overactive conscience.

COGNITIVE THEORY

In cognitive-developmental theory which originated with Piaget (1932) the emphasis has been on children's social-inferential abilities as a prerequisite for prosocial behavior. The young child is viewed as egocentric, assuming that others think and feel the same way s/he does. A certain level of intellectual growth or maturation thus is necessary before the child becomes capable of understanding another's point of view and hence of being altruistic. This approach produced many studies in which children's abilities to take others' social roles or perspectives and their abilities to reason about moral issues were examined in relation to prosocial actions. The assumptions were that the ability (a) to interpret accurately another's needs or (b) to attain a high level (stage) of moral reasoning was necessary for a child to show concern reflected in actual behavior. The results of these research projects are mixed (see reviews by Radke-Yarrow, Zahn-Waxler and Chapman 1983; Shantz 1983) with no strong evidence for the hypothesized connection between social-cognitive capacities and altruistic acts. In other words, one can understand the nature of another's distress without doing anything about it and one can behave in a caring way without highly developed cognitive capacities.

In both psychoanalytic and cognitive theories, there is a long period of early development in which self-concern is presumed to predominate: Consideration for others would not be expected from children until they were at least five to seven years old. Two other theories, ethological/evolutionary and learning theories, do not highlight a particular age or stage of development necessary for altruism to occur. They are considered in greater detail throughout this chapter because of their special relevance to humane education: The ethological approach because it provides an evolutionary perspective and identifies those attributes that we have in common with others (human and animal) and the learning approach because it begins to identify specific mechanisms by which empathy and altruism can be taught and learned.

LEARNING THEORY

In learning theory, the emphasis has been more on the overt, observable prosocial behavior of the child rather than on reasoning and inner motives. In initial formulations, prosocial behavior was presumed to be acquired in the same way as other learned behaviors—through processes of conditioning reinforcement, and modeling (see Radke-Yarrow, Zahn-Waxler, and Chapman 1983). Over time, conceptions of learning were expanded to include the influence of other socialization processes (e.g., nature of parental discipline; specific instruction; institutionalized, cultural norms and so on). For example, different cultures and subcultures have quite different norms that are communicated to the child about cooperative, individualistic and competitive behaviors and what is appropriate balance between them (Madsen and Shapira 1977). Learned norms of responsibility (i.e., that it is our duty to help) and norms of reciprocity (i.e., "I'll help you if you help me") are thought to be culturally determined and learned in institutional settings (school, church, home, etc.).

The values of society impinge most directly on young children through their parent's attitudes and philosophies about moral and altruistic behaviors as well as through their specific teaching and caregiving practices. Some of these practices include (a) what caregivers model or convey in their own behavior about empathy and altruism, (b) what they preach about consideration for others, (c) their general nurturance or warmth toward the child and their own empathy when the child is distressed, (d) their teaching and control practices, when their children cause distress to another (e.g., physical punishment, love withdrawal, explanation and reasoning) (e) the use of praise and punishment, (f) the use of attributions (such as "you are mother's good helper"), and (g) the creation of environments that promote prosocial behavior or make caring possible. Generalizations or formulas for how to produce a prosocial child are difficult and sometimes hazardous, but the bulk of evidence implicates the following caregiver variables as important—the modeling of altruism to others, nurturance toward the child, use of reasoning (and firm discipline when the child hurts others), direct instruction in how to help, and reinforcement for helping (Eisenberg 1983; Radke-Yarrow, Zahn-Waxler and Chapman 1983). In later sections we will consider in greater detail how some of these variables influence the development of empathy and altruism in children. Another approach to the socialization question has been taken by investigators who have examined parental and societal factors that promote or inhibit aggression rather than prosocial behavior. A brief overview of these findings indicates that parental permissiveness and inconsistency are associated with high levels of aggression in their children; also predictive of cruelty in childhood are high levels of parental aggression and abusiveness, both toward the children and others as well (see Parke and Slaby 1983, for a detailed review of this literature). The learning/socialization perspective holds special promise for humane education because it can identify processes that may be alterable and hence may enhance the child's prosocial tendencies.

BIOLOGICAL THEORIES

Ethological/evolutionary approaches, on the other hand, hold promise for understanding the biological bases of altruism and possibly for understanding empathic relationships between humans and animals. In this view, altruism is built into species and some forms of altruism are adaptive for survival. Ethologists emphasize the fact that humans like other animals, are born with behavioral and emotional tendencies that enhance their own likelihood of survival and hence the continuation of the species. Even though human infants are more helpless than the young of any other mammalian species, they are well equipped with reflexes and behaviors of significance for survival (e.g., rooting, sucking, clinging, following). The distress cries of infants are present at the moment of birth: They provide for very effective means of eliciting attention, sympathy, help, and comfort from adults. In all mammals this distress cry or isolation call is a stimulus for caregiving and comfort. It served originally to maintain social cohesion by maintaining maternal-offspring contact. The distress cry of mammals is also a constant reminder that animals other than ourselves do have feelings and are capable of suffering.

There are many characteristics that humans have in common with other mammals that may contribute to maintenance of social contact and hence, possibly, to the development of empathy as well (e.g., social play, nursing, separation distress). Distress is a universal emotion expressed across all mammalian species. Distress is also a stimulus for acts of altruism. It has the potential for evoking an emotional, possibly empathic, response in some other members of the same species. If there is sufficient similarity in expressions of distress across *different* mammalian species, this may be a powerful biological mechanism reminding us that some of the distresses and needs of other species are similar to our own. This recognition of communality might help to promote empathy across species. There is little or no research designed to explore humans' reactions to the cries of other animals. In one of our studies (Zahn-Waxler, Friedman, and Cummings 1983) preschool and elementary school-age children overheard cries of premature and normal babies. It was not uncommon for children initially to mistake the cries, particularly those of the less developed, premature infants, for cries of animals and birds (sheep, donkeys, cats, goats, even kangaroos and turkeys). This did not deter the children from expressing empathy toward the infants with unusual (animal-like) cries. Distress cries, however, should be seen as a necessary but not sufficient condition for eliciting empathy. There are also studies to indicate that distress cries elicit aggressive behavior in some caregivers. Physical abuse and neglect of distressed offspring have been reported in primates as well as humans.

MacLean (1982) has hypothesized that the capacity of mammals for nurturant caregiving toward their (distressed) offspring, in contrast to some reptilians who may abandon or eat their young, is the evolutionary forerunner to the development of empathy, conscience, and a sense of social responsibility. MacLean has attempted to identify those parts of the brain that are responsible for this caregiving. The limbic system is clearly basic for parental care and family affiliation in mammals. But the development of the prefrontal neocortex which is a much more recently evolved structure, has contributed to further development of the family, especially in primates. The added sector of neocortex gives human beings a capacity for foresight, which is believed to underlie our striving for the welfare of our own progeny and the progeny of others. Some scientists also have begun to speculate about neurochemical and hormonal bases of empathy and altruism and the brain circuitry that might be involved (Panksepp, in press).

RESEARCH ON THE DEVELOPMENT OF GENERALIZED ALTRUISM

Many of the processes that explain the origins and development of altruism are difficult to study directly. However, it is possible to study developmentally young children's responses to other's distress cries and hence examine their early capacities for empathy and caregiving. Such research has established the importance of both instinct and environment in the development of sensitivity to another's distress. Studies from the early 1900's demonstrated the possibility that even newborns may be predisposed to be receptive to distress; they are likely to cry, reflexively when they hear the cries of other babies. It was not clear, however, from these studies, whether children cried because they were empathic or because they were frightened or because the sounds of the crier were aversive and painful. More recent and experimentally sophisticated research designs (Simner 1971; Sagi and Hoffman 1976) have confirmed that there is special sensitivity to the cry, per se, and not just to the noisiness of the cry.

We have engaged in two kinds of studies of the development of altruism and empathy in over 175 young children. We have examined the origins and transitions (in one to two-and-a-half year olds) in prosocial patterns over time in natural settings (Zahn-Waxler and Radke-Yarrow 1982); and we have created different learning environments to determine which are most conducive to developing prosocial behavior based on concern for another's welfare (in three to five year olds) (Yarrow, Scott and Waxler 1973). In both studies we have been interested in how children respond to others in *distress*, because this represents the set of conditions most likely to evoke emotion (and hence possibly empathy and altruism). Both kinds of studies explore conditions that create generalized consideration for the welfare of others (i.e., caring for nonfamily as well as family members, for animals as well as humans).

THE EARLY DEVELOPMENT AND SOCIALIZATION OF ALTRUISM

A longitudinal study of one to two-and-a-half year olds examined children's responses to compelling distress situations. A sample of middle-class mothers was trained by research assistants to make systematic, narrative accounts and to tape record their observation reports. The mothers observed events of naturally occurring distress (e.g., pain, sadness, anger) that were either caused or witnessed by the children. This was done over a period of many months. Standard emotional incidents were also introduced. Each week either the mother or a home visitor acted out a distress emotion in the home. These procedures provided thousands of incidents which were then analyzed to determine (a) developmental changes in children's reactions to other's distress and (b) parental socialization practices that were more or less likely to produce altruism. Several hundred of these incidents involved reports of children's feelings and behaviors toward animals.

There are very distinct age changes in how children react to another's distress during the second year of life (Zahn-Waxler and Radke-Yarrow 1982). Children almost always are keenly aware of the distress and if they consistently do not notice, one wonders what is wrong. The youngest children are themselves likely to become distressed, in ways similar to the reflexive crying of newborns but not with such full-blow intensity. Just a little past the first year of life, children begin to comfort others in distress. This is a developmental landmark; an aversive experience in another person draws out a concerned, approach response from the child. Children's first prosocial acts are physical interventions: they pat and hug the victims, rub their hurts and so on. Children often begin to seek out guidance, reassurance, and information from their mothers when in these situations. There is also an explosion of prosocial activity at this time. Children's acts of compassion begin to take many different forms: acts of help, sharing, comforting, rescue, distraction, defense/protection, verbal sympathy, are now present in development. These reactions occur not only when children are innocent bystanders to the others' distress (e.g., watching mother stub her toe) but also when they have caused the harm (e.g., biting sister). The first prosocial interventions are largely, as one might expect, confined to family members. If families have pets, the animal sometimes become recipients of the child's first expressions of empathy. We have described the range of prosocial responses to humans elsewhere (Zahn-Waxler and Radke-Yarrow 1982). There is considerable overlap in the ways young children express kindness to animals and people. Table 1 provides illustrations from our data of the different kinds of prosocial behaviors that young children show to animals. And Table 2 provides examples of child's aggressive tendencies toward animals.

Virtually all of the children studied showed this early capacity for concern for the welfare of another being. This *uniformity* suggests that altruism is a biological given, "wired" in and ready for expression given sufficient physical, cognitive, and emotional growth. There were differences among children in the frequency and emotional intensity of

Table 1

Compassionate Behaviors Toward Animals Shown by One-and-a-Half to Two-and-a-Half Year Old Children*

1. Child throws rubber toy at dog. Mother says, "Oh, you've hurt Bruno, poor Bruno." Child reaches over and hugs dog around the neck, then lies down on the hearth with the dog.

2. The dog begins to gasp for breath: Child runs over and smiled at first. Then he looks serious and throws himself on the dog to console him. Mother encourages him to get off. Mother comforts the dog by stroking its head and neck, and the child pats too.

3. Child pulls the dog's foot hard and the dog yelps. Mother says, "Oh, don't pull Suzy's foot like that." Child looks serious, touches foot and says "hurt." Mother becomes very excited because this is the first time child has used a word that expresses a feeling. She says, "Yes, it did hurt, but it doesn't anymore." Child then pats dog's paw very lovingly and gently, and hugs the dog.

4. Cat gets caught in the window well and girl cries with concern.

5. Dog sneezes and child brings Kleenex to blow its nose.

6. A dead goldfinch lies on the doorstep. Child points and said, "Birdie, birdie." and keeps looking at it with a furrowed brow—kind of sad-like.

7. The dog comes in making little crying sounds. The child turns around and says very sympathetically, "What's the matter, Lady? What's the matter?"

8. Mother is rough housing with the dog and hits a sore spot. He yelps, the mother tries to console and the girl comforts the dog as well.

9. Child steps on the dog's foot and he gave a snappy growl. Mother grabbed the dog, yelled at him and threw him in the basement. Father joined in. Child squawks back at parents in a loud harsh tone, i.e., she came to the defense of the dog by scolding her parents for yelling at the dog.

10. Child starts hitting the cat and pulls its tail. Mother moves child away and says, "No, we do not do that to cats, not at all. We treat them nicely. We never pull their tails and we never kick them." Then child begins to pat and kiss the cat.

11. Child is eating a snack and tries to share her animal crackers with the dog.

12. Child pulls dog's ears and dog gives a high little squeak. Mother notes that child doesn't seem to realize that those are squeaks of pain. So she has to tell him, "No, don't hurt the doggie; be gentle." Then he puts his arms around the dog's neck, puts his cheek to the dog's head and is sweet and gentle. (On another occasion like this, the mother explains but also slaps the child thus giving a mixed message.)

*Excerpted from mothers' observational records.

their altruism. This *variability* might result, in part, from differences in what children are being taught by their parents about responsiveness to the needs of others.

We examined three aspects of child-rearing and socialization that might be expected to influence young children's orientations to others in distress (Zahn-Waxler, Radke-Yarrow and King 1979). One concerns the nurturance or warmth of the caregiver and the sensitivity

Table 2

Aggressive or Callous Behaviors Toward Animals Shown by One-and-a-Half to Two-and-a-Half Year-Old Children*

1. Mother calls the dog who won't come and mother says, "That dumb dog!" Child mimics mother's tone and says, "Get in here dumb dog."
2. Father is "real harsh" with the dog and the child, in turn, starts to berate the dog—yelling at him in the same kind of tone of voice.
3. Dog gets into chicken livers. Mother yells loudly, "Get down and get out of here dog," smacks him and shoos him out of the kitchen. A few minutes later the dog comes back in and the child imitates the mother, waving her arms, yelling at and hitting the dog.
4. Dog chokes and child laughs hilariously.
5. Child is squeezing a kitten's neck. Mother is worried that he might be able to hurt it. So she wraps her hands around the child's neck, to give him the idea of how unpleasant it is to have one's neck squeezed. He drops the kitten and she stopped squeezing.
6. Mother fusses at the dog. Child goes up to the dog, stomps her foot, jabbers to him—really trying to tell him off, calling him "Bad" and so on.

*Excerpted from mother's observational records.

with which s/he handles the child when the child is distressed. This is one kind of index of the parent's empathy toward the child. Also, important are the parent's teachings and emotional reactions when parent and child view someone who is hurt or upset. For example, does the parent model altruism to the victim by helping, consoling, and so on, does s/he reassure the child, or does s/he ignore the situation entirely? The parent also plays a significant role when the child causes distress. Children's acts of aggression (e.g., hitting father, pulling the cat's tail) provide further occasions for teaching. Caregivers may use a variety of techniques here, sometimes in combination. These include for example, (a) power assertion (physical punishment or restraint), (b) withdrawal of love (e.g., sending the child to his room or coldly ignoring him), (c) verbal prohibitions ("stop it!"), (d) suggesting a positive, alternative behavior ("why don't you pet kitty instead of pulling on him?"), (e) reasoning or explanations about the consequences for the other ("you make Joey feel bad when you take his toy"; "that hurts Blacky when you step on his paw"), (f) perspective-taking, "Remember what it felt like when your foot got caught?", and (g) ignoring the situation. Some of these parental techniques are also illustrated in Table 1.

The content (or substance) of children's prosocial actions often appeared to have been learned (imitated) from the parents' own actions (e.g., mother shows child how to pat gently, or put on a Band-Aid). A very major parental influence had to do with the ways in which children were disciplined for hurting others. Mothers who had the most prosocial children used the following techniques: (1) They gave clear explanations about the negative consequences for the victim when the child hurt others; (2) they were sometimes moralistic and judgmental ("it's not nice to bite"; "I don't want to be near you when you act like that"); (3) they provided their children with general rules about physical aggression toward people and animals ("you must never hurt others"); and (4) they firmly prohibited their children from hurting others in specific situations and suggested positive, alternative actions. The children were more likely to make reparation for distresses they had caused and to come to the aid of victims they had not themselves harmed. Mothers who used this constellation of disciplinary techniques also tended to be highly empathic and sensitive to the needs of their own children when they themselves experienced distress.

The strong relationships between maternal practices and early child (prosocial) behaviors suggests that this is a time in the child's life when there is special receptivity and sensitivity to environmental influences, and hence to teachings about kindness toward others. A follow-up study of these families five years later showed that those children who showed high levels of generalized altruism and remorse over hurting others as toddlers were also the more altruistic children by the time they entered school (Cummings et. al., in press). Thus, we must take seriously the possibility that basic humane attitudes and behaviors are laid down in the first years of life and teachings can begin then. Young children can be made to understand that animals as well as people, have feelings, are receptive to affection, and sometimes require consolation.

Children's imitations of parental behaviors were by no means restricted to parents' prosocial actions (e.g., see Table 2). In at least half of the families studied, parents showed anger to animals and children imitated parent's expressions of anger and disciplinary action. This included episodes of shouting at and hitting animals. Sometimes we would see the young child embellish the parent's punitive action by yelling and hitting when the parent had just shouted. In some families, this appeared to be part of a consistent pattern. For example, one mother described an incident in which she yelled at the dog, picked him by the collar and "sort of" threw him down. In her words—"I get very violent with him because he really annoys me sometimes; I think I even kicked him." She noted that usually when she does this her one-year-old becomes frightened or angry too, but this time that didn't happen. Perhaps the child was already developing defensive coping strategies. We also saw the other extreme—families where pets were treated with respect and accorded family status. In such homes, children were often unusually responsive to the plights of pets. In one family, when the dog sneezed, the two-year-old boy would bring a kleenex to blow its nose, and when the dog hiccupped, the child tenderly kissed its nose. When the mother brushed the dog and hair came out, the boy interpreted it as a hurt and tried to shield the dog from the mother while anxiously attempting to pat the hair back on.

Humane and inhumane orientations of children thus may derive from the values fostered and the treatment of animals provided within the family. We have identified some of the parental practices that may promote compassion and dampen aggression. We found that mothers' communications about the need for humane behavior occur most frequently and with special intensity when their young children are themselves harming others. However, in another study of preschool children we found that young children can also be taught to help when they are bystanders to another's distress. An experimental research approach was used. Different learning environments were created to determine what kind of caregiver practices were most likely to produce generalized altruism in bystander circumstances.

THE TEACHING OF GENERALIZED ALTRUISM

Four experimental environments were developed to represent configurations of rearing conditions that differed in the adult's nurturant relationship with the child, and in how she conveyed her own prosocial principles, feelings, and behavior. The children were from middle-class and upper-middle-class families. They were assigned to nursery school groups in which an adult provided either highly nurturant or relatively aloof, matter-of-fact care. These experimental conditions took place in 30-minute periods in the nursery school over a period of two weeks. Following these "histories of rearing" the adult provided one of two kinds of programmed experiences that dealt with prosocial content. In type "A" conditions, the adult expressed prosocial principles and values in relation to many incidents of distress presented in pictures and in miniature play materials (dioramas depicting a child, an adult, or an animal in some kind of situation in which help was needed). The adult's reactions to these symbolized distresses combined inductive reasoning, positive emotional involvement, modeling of help, and provision of information. Thus, she explained, "Look, this little bunny is caught in the bush and can't get out. Poor bunny must be scared. I am going to help it out of the bush so it can get back to its mother. There, that makes the bunny feel better." The child would then have a turn at helping. Type "B" conditions included the preceding procedures, with the important addition of the adult's responding similarly to programmed distresses that involved interaction with real people and animals (e.g., a teacher dropping her pencils, a cat tangled in yarn, etc.). These training conditions took place over several weeks. Both sets of rearing techniques provided the child with information intended to help the child to recognize cues of distress and feelings of the victim; to demonstrate ways of helping, and to indicate the consequences of such helping for the victim. The "A" and "B" procedures differed in two important respects: (1) Principles expressed by the adult in A conditions were only at the level of the hypothetical or abstract; in B conditions principles were put into practice with real consequences for the distressed persons. (2) Prosocial modeling by the adult in B conditions involved interaction with the distressed person which gave the adult the direct experience of the consequences of her prosocial interventions. High and low nurturant histories were used with each training type. These four conditions were intended as a study of configurations of rearing conditions as they are practiced in real life by parents and experienced by children. All four conditions resulted in more symbolic altruism than the control condition where no forms of teaching were done. One of the four configurations of rearing conditions produced a significantly higher frequency of real helping behavior from the children and more verbal expressions of sympathetic feelings than the other three conditions. It was an adult with whom the child had a history of a nurturant relationship and who provided the child with the model of her own caring behavior for others in both symbolic and real interactions with those in need. Also, in this condition, the adult's prosocial interactions involved child, adult and animal victims of distress and has clear cognitive and positive affective accompaniments. The adult provided the child with information about the victim's experience, the adult's own feelings, and the consequences of her prosocial intervention. The same set of rearing conditions that produced the highest levels of altruism in these children was similarly effective with a group of lower-class children in a replication study (Yarrow, Scott and Waxler 1973).

If we were to generalize from these experimental findings to child-rearing in the real world, we would conclude that the parent who is altruistic toward others but is cold with his child is not going to have much success in developing generalized altruism in his child. Further, the parent who conveys his moral values as principles only, but does not translate these into real, caring actions, accomplishes a similar limited kind of learning in the child. Generalized altruism appears to be best learned from parents who both inculcate the principles and show real altruism in their everyday interactions. And their practices toward their children are consistent with their general altruism.

SUMMARY AND CONCLUSIONS

Our research provides substantial evidence of empathy and altruism in children at ages well before many theories would have it occur. The tendencies of young children sometimes to be egocentric, dependent, lacking in competence, demanding, narcissistic, and so on, have been emphasized in many theories of personality and cognitive development. Hence, we have been inclined to ignore their tender, prosocial side and the fact that they do have considerable social skills. Also contributing to an inaccurate view of young children as very limited in their empathic capacities are the research methods used. Cognitive/developmental studies often rely on interviews of children and this puts young children at a particular disadvantage. Often they cannot put into words the reasons for their acts of caring, they cannot state abstract principles of justice, and they evidence primitive, unsophisticated verbal understanding of moral issues. They then become labelled as functioning at a low stage of moral development, and are stereotyped as hedonistic, exploitative, negativistic, dominionistic, and so on in their orientations toward others. These characterizations are based on poorly applied understanding of young children's words rather than on their deeds and their expressed emotions.

While some studies report that children become more prosocial with age, many other studies of cooperation, comforting, helping, and sharing do not show the expected age increase (Radke-Yarrow, Zahn-Waxler and Chapman 1983). The research situations in which older children have been shown to be more likely than younger children to manifest prosocial behavior are research situations in which the victim's plight is portrayed symbolically and children must share with a hypothetical other (i.e., as in giving to charity). Older children will necessarily be better able to understand such abstractions and representations of distress and will have developed greater competencies for prosocial behavior that requires these abilities. This does not mean, however, that children necessarily develop a greater emotional capacity for empathy as they grow older. In fact, the opposite sometimes may be true for many because they have had more time to learn other values and practices, to treat distress as routine, and to have developed defenses for shutting out their own and others pain. It is reasonable to assume that children of all ages are capable of learning to be kind. The ways in which they learn will differ considerably. This is an area where much research is needed to help plan the most effective curricula for children of different ages.

Our research is not unique in finding that young children's capacities for concerned feelings and behaviors far outstrip their verbal competencies. Increasingly, there are studies that corroborate the occurrence, in the first years of life, of children's understanding of others' inner feelings; children's abilities to cooperate, take turns with others, and negotiate conflicts, show willingness to share with peers and adults, and manifest capabilities for giving help (e.g., Bretherton, McNew and Beeghley-Smith 1981; Eckerman, Whatley and Kutz 1975; Rheingold, Hay and West 1976; Ross and Goldmam 1977; Hay and Ross 1982). These findings are not merely an academic issue. They influence whether we view young children as altruistic or hedonistic, and determine when, if, and how we will attempt to teach them compassionate behavior. Our data, and those of others, indicate that training should begin very early and that it should recognize the child's innate empathic sensitivies. It is commonly recommended that children be at least five to six years old before they are allowed to have pets because this is when they can first begin to assume some real responsibility. This decision precludes exposure to animals in those important early years of life where basic orientations are established.

The research has specific implications for curricula that are designed to develop and encourage empathic and humane behavior in young children. The following factors have been found to be important: (a) having warm and accepting relationships with the parent/teacher if the learning is to generalize, (b) using training materials that realistically portray feelings and distress, (c) giving the child direct experience with real helping, (d) beginning teaching very early in the child's life and making it a family affair, (e) using explicit explanations about feelings and circumstances of the victim, i.e., actively evoking empathy in the child, and (f) stating general codes or principles about altruism, aggression, and morality, in simple, explicit terms. Many of these notions are probably already part of existing curricula and hence may represent what is already conventional wisdom to some. To large numbers of people, however, it is not common knowledge that empathy and humane behavior can be taught and learned even in the earliest years of life.

To summarize, as early as the second year of life, one can begin to teach children the rudiments of a sense of responsibility for other people and animals. This teaching task should continue through childhood, with an attempt both to retain the child's early empathic proclivities and to be sensitive to the changing cognitive and symbolic capacities that occur with development. It is possible to show even young children specific ways of helping and caring for others. The verbal messages and the physical demonstrations of appropriate actions need to be simple, direct, concrete, consistent, and repeated in a variety of contexts throughout the early years of life. It is especially important with toddlers and preschoolers (and with older children as well) that the teaching not always be at an abstract symbolic levels, (i.e., with pictures, stories, teddy bears, etc.) Rather, "hands on" experiences with real animals and persons, with their needs, their discomforts, and the specific caretaking they require will be necessary to equip children with the knowledge and motivation for responding humanely.

The mothers' reports in the longitudinal study of altruism provided us with many detailed narrative records of family interaction with pets. Based on clinical evaluations of these reports we offer the following observations and generalizations. Many of the families had pets but there was considerable variability in the ways in which animals were incorporated into the family and in their specific roles and functions. Parents vary considerably in how much they praise and reward children's nurturing of animals and how much teasing they tolerate. Some parents find the child's abuse or aggression "cute" while others firmly apprise their children of the distress this creates for the animal. There are differences (described earlier) in the techniques parents use to prevent the child from hurting and encourage the child to be more caring. Hence, parents presumably differ in the extent to which they believe animals have feelings, are receptive to affection, and require comfort.

Some parents clearly use pets as the scapegoats for other family and personal problems: in volatile, angry families, animals are the recipients of displaced aggression, receiving more than their share of hostility for minor misdeeds. Some of the parents give mixed messages to their children about the value of the pets and the children, in turn, reflect this ambivalence in their own treatment of animals. Thus, they can be seen to alternate between affection and abuse, with little awareness of this inconsistency in their treatment. The research literature and common sense would lead us to expect that children will learn to be caring, or abusive, or indifferent to animals depending on whether they see the parent behave in a similar way. It is more complicated, however. Some children may be relatively unresponsive to parental teachings and some may react against their parents. One little girl, for example, sided with the animal in situations of conflict and consistently tried to protect it against parental punishment, sometimes literally putting herself in the middle. This kind of compassion (i.e., early adoption of the defender role) thus may have very different origins from the compassion based on positive teachings. Even if families have pets early in child's life, this does not assure a good learning situation. There is considerable variability in early family experiences with animals; children will come to early training and education programs with very different attitudes, behavior styles, values, and emotional orientations toward animals. These patterns may already be pervasive and entrenched. Teaching techniques then will have to be adapted to reach each child.

It is interesting to speculate concerning why domestic cats and dogs evolved. Mostly, we take them for granted but they are an anomaly in the animal kindgom in terms of (a) their propensity to form more intense social attachments outside of their own species (i.e., to humans) than within it, and (b) their ability to elicit strong expressions of affect from humans. These mutual attachments were thought to have evolved originally because cats and dogs were useful to human physical survival,—in keeping down the rodent population, in protecting, and defending humans, and so on. Yet, even when these needs no longer existed, people continued to have pets, perhaps more to fill psychological and emotional needs. The extensive recent use of pets as "therapists" attest to their remarkable capacity for reducing stress and providing companionship, comfort, and pleasure to others (Katcher and Beck 1983). We make animals an important part of children's lives from infancy onward. As babies they are given stuffed animals of all kinds and many of their first experiences with comfort (given and received) are with these play objects. The first dreams of children are reported to have more animal than human themes. Also, many early educational materials make use of animal characters. Some people believe that there is a natural, special affinity or empathic bond between young children and animals (though there is the potential for cruelty as well). We have many reasons for giving pets to children. Pets provide companionship and comfort, they provide an opportunity for less ambivalent emotional relationships, they may help to ameliorate family tensions. Some mothers, for example, indicate that the child goes to the family's cat or dog for comfort after having been disciplined. Animals also provide an opportunity to learn to be responsible for others, to be gentle, and to discipline effectively. Because the life span of a pet is often shorter than the periods of childhood and adolescence of humans, children's first experiences with suffering, death and mourning, issues of mortality and immortality often will be in relation to their pets. Thus, animals provide an arena for teaching and learning (at both cognitive and emotional levels) about many of the major issues and struggles basic to existence.

Darwin's travels and observations led him to reaffirm, as have others before and after him, that man is not the center of the universe. Man is connected to a larger web of life. We are a fellow species who need to share the earth with other species. Family pets may serve a very special purpose of reminding us of this connection between human life and animal life and the emotional needs we have in common with other animals.

Many of the issues that concern us here are conveyed with eloquence and insight in de Saint-Exupéry's book, *The Little Prince* (1943). The prince, a young boy, travels to many planets, and talks to many people in his quest to know about the meaning of life. At last, on earth, he learns from a fox what is important. The boy meets a wild fox one morning and invites him to play. The fox tells the prince he cannot play with him because he is not yet tame. The prince asks what it means to tame and the fox replies, "It is an act too often neglected. It means to establish ties. Until we establish ties, neither of us is special to each other. But if you tame me, then we shall need each other. To me you will be unique in all the world. To you, I will be unique in all the world,"—"You become responsible forever for what you have tamed." The fox teaches the boy how to tame him and they form a close bond. Eventually they must part and the fox is about to cry. The prince speculates that it might have been better never to have met because of the pain of separation. The fox assures the prince that it is infinitely better to have formed the relationship because through the process, they have become unique in all the world. It is this complex and poorly understood process of relationship formation, whether between people or between people and animals, that helps to foster empathy and diminish aggression.

REFERENCES

Bretherton, I., McNew, S., and Beeghley-Smith, M. 1981. Early person knowledge as expressed in gestural and verbal communications: When do infants acquire a "theory of mind?" In: *Infant social cognition.* Hillsdale, New Jersey: Lawrence Erlbaum Associates.

Burleson, B.R. *Comforting communication. Understanding interpersonal communication: Social cognitive strategic processes in children and adults.* Beverly Hills, California: Sage, in press.

Cummings, M., Zahn-Waxler, C., Iannotti, R.J., Hollenbeck, B., and Radke-Yarrow, M. Early organization of altruism and aggression: Developmental patterns and individual differences. In: Zahn-Waxler, C., Cummings, E.M., and Iannotti, R.J. eds. *Altruism and aggression, social and biological origins.* Cambridge Press, in press.

de Saint Exupéry, A. 1943. *The Little Prince.* New York: Harcourt, Brace and Javanovitch.

Dymond, R.F. 1945. A preliminary investigation of the relation of insight and empathy. *Journal of Consulting Psychology* 12(4):228–33.

Eckerman, C.O., Whatley, J.L., and Kutz, S.L. 1975. Growth of social play with peers during the second year of life. *Developmental Psychology* 11:42–49.

Eisenberg, N. 1983. The socialization and development of empathy and prosocial behavior. The Humane Society of the United States, Fort Worth, Texas, October 1983. Symposium: *Can love be taught: Animals, empathy and education.*

Feshbach, S. and Feshbach, N. Altruism and aggression: A personality perspective. In: Zahn-Waxler, C., Cummings, E.M., and Iannotti, R.J. eds., *Altruism and aggression: Social and biological origins.* Cambridge Press, in press.

Hay, D.F. and Ross, H.S. 1982. The social nature of early conflict. *Child Development* 53:105–13.

Hoffman, M.L. 1975. Empathy, role-taking, guilt, and the development of altruistic motives. In:Likona, T. ed. *Moral development and behavior.* New York: Holt, Rinehart, and Winston.

Hogan, R. 1973. Moral conduct and moral character: A psychological perspective. *Psychological Bulletin* 79(4):217–32.

Katcher, A.H. and Beck, A.M. 1983. eds. *New perspectives on our lives with companion animals.* Philadelphia: University of Pennsylvania Press.

MacLean, P. 1982. *Evolutionary brain roots of family, play, and the isolation call.* The Adolph Meyer Lecture, 135th Annual Meeting of the American Psychiatric Association, Toronto, Canada, May 18.

Madsen, M.C. and Shapira, A. 1977. Cooperation and challenge in four cultures. *Journal of Social Psychology* 102:189–95.

Meade, G.H. 1934. *Mind, self, and society.* Chicago: University of Chicago Press.

Miller, N.E. 1983. Understanding the use of animals in behavioral research: Some critical issues. In:Sechzer, J.A. ed. *The role of animals in biomedical research. Annals of the New York Academy of Sciences,* Vol. 406:113–8.

Olinick, S.L. 1980. *The psychotherapeutic instrument.* New York: Aronson.

Panksepp, J. The psychobiology of prosocial behaviors: Separation distress, play and altruism. In:Zahn-Waxler, C., Cummings, E.M., and Iannotti, R.H. eds. *Altruism and aggression: Social and biological origins.* Cambridge Press, in press.

Parke, R.D. and Slaby, R.G. 1983. The development of aggression. In:Mussen, P.H. ed. *Carmichael's manual of child psychology* (Vol. IV, 4th ed., Hetherington, H., ed.) New York: John Wiley and Sons.

Piaget, J. 1965. *The moral judgment of the child.* Glencoe, Ill.: Free Press. (originally published, 1932).

Radke-Yarrow, M., Zahn-Waxler, C., and Chapman, M. Children's prosocial dispositions and behavior. In:Mussen, P.H. ed. *Carmichael's manual of child psychology* (Vol. IV, 4th ed., Hetherington, E., ed.), New York: John Wiley and Sons, pp. 469-546.

Rheingold, H., Hay, D., and West, M. 1976. Sharing in the second year of life. *Child Development* 47:1148-58.

Rogers, C.R. 1957. The necessary and sufficient conditions of therapeutic personality change. *Journal of Consulting Psychology* 21:95-103.

Ross, H.S. and Goldman, B.D. 1977. Establishing new social relations in infancy. In:Alloway, T., Krames, L. and Plinar, P. eds. *Advances in communication and affect.* Vol. 4. New York: Plenum Press.

Sagi, A. and Hoffman, M.L. 1976. Empathic distress in the newborn. *Developmental Psychology* 12:175-6.

Shantz, C.U. 1983. Social cognition. In:Mussen, P.H. ed. *Carmichael's manual of child psychology*, (Vol. III, 4th ed.), Flavell, J.H. and Markman, E.M. eds. New York: John Wiley and Sons.

Simner, M.L. 1971. Newborn's response to the cry of another infant. *Developmental Psychology* 5:136-50.

Wilson, E.O. 1975. *Sociobiology: The new synthesis.* Cambridge, Mass.: Harvard University Press.

Yarrow, M., Scott, P., and Waxler, C. 1973. Learning concern for others. *Developmental Psychology* 8:240-60.

Zahn-Waxler, C., and Radke-Yarrow, M. 1982. The development of altruism: Alternative research strategies. In:Eisenberg, N. ed. *The development of prosocial behavior.* New York: Academic Press. pp. 109-37.

Zahn-Waxler, C., Radke-Yarrow, M., and King, R. 1979. Child rearing and children's prosocial initiations toward victims of distress. *Child Development* 50:319-30.

ATTITUDES TOWARD ANIMALS: AGE-RELATED DEVELOPMENT AMONG CHILDREN*

Stephen R. Kellert**

School of Forestry and Environmental Studies,
Yale University
New Haven, Connecticut 06511

Abstract

This paper reviews the results of a study of 267 children in the 2nd, 5th, 8th, and 11th grades. A battery of tests was used to examine children's knowledge and attitudes towards animals, and behavioral contacts with animals. A typology of basic attitudes towards animals and appropriate scales was employed. Children's knowledge and attitudes towards animals were also compared to those of adults 18 years of age and over. Major differences occurred among children distinguished by age, sex, ethnicity, and urban/rural residence. Additionally, significant knowledge and attitude variations occurred among diverse animal-related activity groups (e.g., among children who hunted, birdwatched, learned about animals in school). Perhaps the most important finding was the identification of three stages in the development of children's perceptions of animals. The transition from

*This study was funded by grants from the U.S. Fish and Wildlife Service and G.R. Dodge Foundation. For details of Dr. Kellert's earlier and more extensive study of American attitudes toward and knowledge of animals, see *Appendix.*

**Many thanks to Miriam Westervelt who co-authored the U.S. Fish and Wildlife Service, General Printing Office report #024-010-00641-2 of the children's study.

6 to 9 years of age primarily involved major changes in affective, emotional relationships to animals. The change from 10 to 13 years of age was marked by a major increase in cognitive, factual understanding and knowledge of animals. The shift from 13 to 16 years of age witnessed a dramatic broadening in ethical concern and ecological appreciation of animals and the natural environment.

INTRODUCTION

This report is the fifth in a series of studies on American attitudes, knowledge and behaviors toward animals and natural habitats. The first three reports focused on the findings of a national survey of 3, 107 adult Americans residing in the 48 contiguous states and Alaska (Kellert 1979, 1980a; Kellert and Berry 1981). The fourth report considered historical trends in American animal use and perception during the twentieth century (Kellert and Westervelt 1982). This fifth report focuses on children's attitudes, knowledge and behaviors toward animals.

Children's perceptions of animals, particularly very young children, are especially difficult to study (Pomerantz 1977). This study should, therefore, be regarded as exploratory, preliminary and tentative. Because of its exploratory character, this study did not include a random sample of American children. The sample was instead confined to the state of Connecticut, although representative numbers of children from each age, sex, urban/rural, and black/white category were included. The total sample included 63 second, 68 fifth, 67 eighth, and 69 eleventh grade students: a total of 267 children. Because somewhat similar methodologies were employed in the study of adult Americans, the children's sample will at times be compared with results obtained in the national adult survey.

KNOWLEDGE OF ANIMALS

Knowledge of animals was assessed primarily in four ways: a series of 33 true/false and multiple choice questions, a pictorial identification test of 15 animals, 11 questions regarding the primary foods of selected animals, and a film test focusing on ecological relationships.

The results generally indicated that most children possessed a limited knowledge of animals. For example, less than 30% of the children were aware that the spring peeper is a frog, and only 29% knew koala bears are not really bears. A disappointing 21% understood veal does not come from lamb, and 55% believed whales are a large fish. A better but disappointing 60% realized all birds do not fly south for the winter, but only 52% knew the penguin is a bird, just 26% knew a tern is not an insect, and only 29% realized tigers do not live in Africa.

Lack of ecological understanding was suggested by responses to the film testing segment. Most children interpreted predation and nutrient cycling in anthropomorphic and negative terms, rarely appreciating or identifying the ecological values of these activities. The efforts of dung beetles were generally considered "disgusting," and many children regarded predation as "wrong."

However, some encouraging knowledge results did emerge. Children as a whole, and 11th graders in particular, were significantly more knowledgeable than adults on questions concerning invertebrates and the basic biological characteristics of animals (Table 1). Adults were, however, more knowledgeable than children about domestic animals and situations involving animals inflicting injury on people and property. Greater knowledge of invertebrates among children was suggested by 78% of all children and 86% of 11th graders, compared to 50% of adults, knowing spiders do not have 10 legs. When adults were compared with 11th graders only, 23% of adults versus 48% of the students knew inch worms are not in the same family as earth worms.

Table 1. Mean correct score by types of knowledge questions

	Children's and adult samples		
	All children (<18 years of age)	11th grade	Adult (<18 years of age)
Biological characteristics	56.8	63.9	55.3
Invertebrates	47.5	51.3	34.7
Human injury	39.5	47.8	63.4
Domestic animals	39.2	44.4	53.4
Taxonomic characteristics	37.3	43.9	38.5
Endangered species	24.6	24.6	27.4

Based on mean scores, children were most knowledgeable about the basic biological characteristics of animals (e.g., "snakes are covered by a thin layer of slime") and invertebrates. These knowledge question categories had overall mean scores, respectively, of 56.8 and 47.5, on a scoring range from 0 to 100. Adults had a dramatically lower invertebrate question mean score of 34.7. The adults, however, obtained a significantly higher mean score on questions concerning human injury or property damage—63.4 versus a children's mean of 39.5. Both children and adults had similar scores on the "taxonomic characteristics of animals" category (e.g., "koala bears are not really bears")—37.3 and 38.5 respectively. Both groups possessed relatively little knowledge of endangered species.

Children were relatively able to recognize a variety of animal species. At least 85% correctly identified a bluejay, swan, rattlesnake, eagle, raccoon, dolphin, wolf and monarch butterfly. Almost three-quarters correctly identified a duck, although only 28% recognized it as a mallard duck. On the other hand, only 8% could identify a great blue heron, just one-third recognized a duck-billed platypus, and only 15% knew a bobwhite.

Children were also knowledgeable about the primary foods of a variety of species. Most children knew what foods were mainly eaten by mice, rabbits, wolves, owls, robins, caterpillers, snakes, and frogs. Only a minority, however, knew which foods were primarily consumed by trout, deer, and bobcats.

Highly significant knowledge scale differences occurred among children distinguished by age, ethnicity, and geographic place of residence. Male/female differences were also significant but at a more modest .02 confidence level (Table 2). Eleventh grade children had the

Table 2. Analysis of variance and multiple classification results on knowledge scale among age, sex, ethnic and urban/rural groups

	Sig F	$\bar{X}$ score	Deviation from grand mean after adjusting for independent and covariate variables
Age	.00		
2nd grade		30.50	−13.99
5th grade		39.64	− 5.64
8th grade		51.18	7.45
11th grade		55.11	11.57
Sex	.02		
Male		47.03	2.47
Female		41.82	− 2.39
Ethnicity	.02		
White		47.40	1.17
Nonwhite		31.60	− 5.72
Urban/rural	.00		
Urban		38.00	− 5.96
Small city		46.90	− 1.13
Suburb		42.90	− 1.13
Rural		52.30	5.23

highest mean scores; 2nd graders, the lowest. Relatively high knowledge scores occurred among rural children and 8th graders. In contrast, relatively low knowledge means were characteristic of black children and children residing in large cities.

Age distinctions were especially impressive. Knowledge scale differences among 8th and 11th graders, however, were substantially less divergent than between 5th and 8th graders, suggesting a decline in the effect of age. An absence of knowledge scale differences among adults over 18 years of age further suggested decreasing importance of age on knowledge of animals.

Ethnic differences were very striking, particularly the very low knowledge scores of nonwhites. Black children had the lowest knowledge scores of any demographic group with the exception of 2nd graders. These knowledge scale differences remained after considering the possible confounding effects of other demographic variables, particularly urban/rural residence.

Urban/rural differences were very significant, particularly when comparing children living in large cities with those residing in the most rural areas. Rural children had the second highest knowledge scale scores, in contrast to children residing in large cities, who had the third lowest scores.

Male/female differences were less pronounced, although still significant at the .02 level. Significantly higher male knowledge scores typically occurred when the animal was a predator. Species preference results also revealed a more negative view of predator animals among female children.

ATTITUDES TOWARD ANIMALS

A typology of basic attitudes toward animals was developed during previous research on adult relationships to animals. Brief definitions of nine attitude types are indicated in Table 3, although more thorough descriptions are available elsewhere (Kellert 1980b). Survey scales were developed to measure each of the attitudes, although it proved impossible to obtain an adequate aesthetic scale. Fifty-four questions were used for measuring the eight attitude scales. Additionally, a 30-minute film, and an accompanying 87-item questionnaire, were created to provide a less structured and more visually sensitive test of attitudes toward animals. Approximately 70 films were reviewed to obtain appropriate segments for this film methodology. The relative independence of the eight attitude scales was suggested by scale intercorrelations of .30 and less with the exception of the

Table 3. Attitudes toward animals

Naturalistic:	Primary interest and affection for wildlife and the outdoors.
Ecologistic:	Primary concern for the environment as a system, for interrelationships between wildlife species and natural habitats.
Humanistic:	Primary interest and strong affection for individual animals, principally pets.
Moralistic:	Primary concern for the right and wrong treatment of animals, with strong opposition to exploitation or cruelty toward animals.
Scientistic:	Primary interest in the physical attributes and biological functioning of animals.
Aesthetic:	Primary interest in the artistic and symbolic characteristics of animals.
Utilitarian:	Primary concern for the practical and material value of animals or the animal's habitat.
Dominionistic:	Primary interest in the mastery and control of animals typically in sporting situations.
***Negativistic:**	Primary orientation an active avoidance of animals due to indifference, dislike or fear.

*Hypothetically, the negativistic attitude can be divided into two attitude types: neutralistic attitude reflecting a passive avoidance of animals due to indifference; and, a negativistic attitude characterized by dislike and fear of animals. In this research, only one encompassing attitude has been considered.

negativistic and naturalistic, and negativistic and ecologistic attitudes, which correlated at the +.48 level.

The relative occurrence of the attitudes was assessed by examining attitude scale score frequency distributions, the slope of the regression line of the frequency distributions, and standardized attitude scale mean scores. According to these indicators, the most common attitude was the humanistic (Figure 1). This attitude scale had the highest mean score, lowest slope figure (indicative of a more dispersed frequency distribution), and included more children in the higher scoring ranges. Also indicative of the relative "popularity" of the humanistic attitude was the finding of "loveable animals" as the most preferred type of animal, cited by 39% of the children (Table 4). In general, strong emotional attachment to individual animals, and a tendency toward anthropomorphism, were the most typical perceptions of animals among the children studied.

The second and third most frequent attitudes were the naturalistic and negativistic. These attitudes were negatively correlated, suggesting two somewhat conflicting perspectives of animals as common among children. The relative "popularity" of the naturalistic perspective was also suggested by "animals in the woods" as the second most

Figure 1: Frequency distributions and mean scores of attitude scales, children

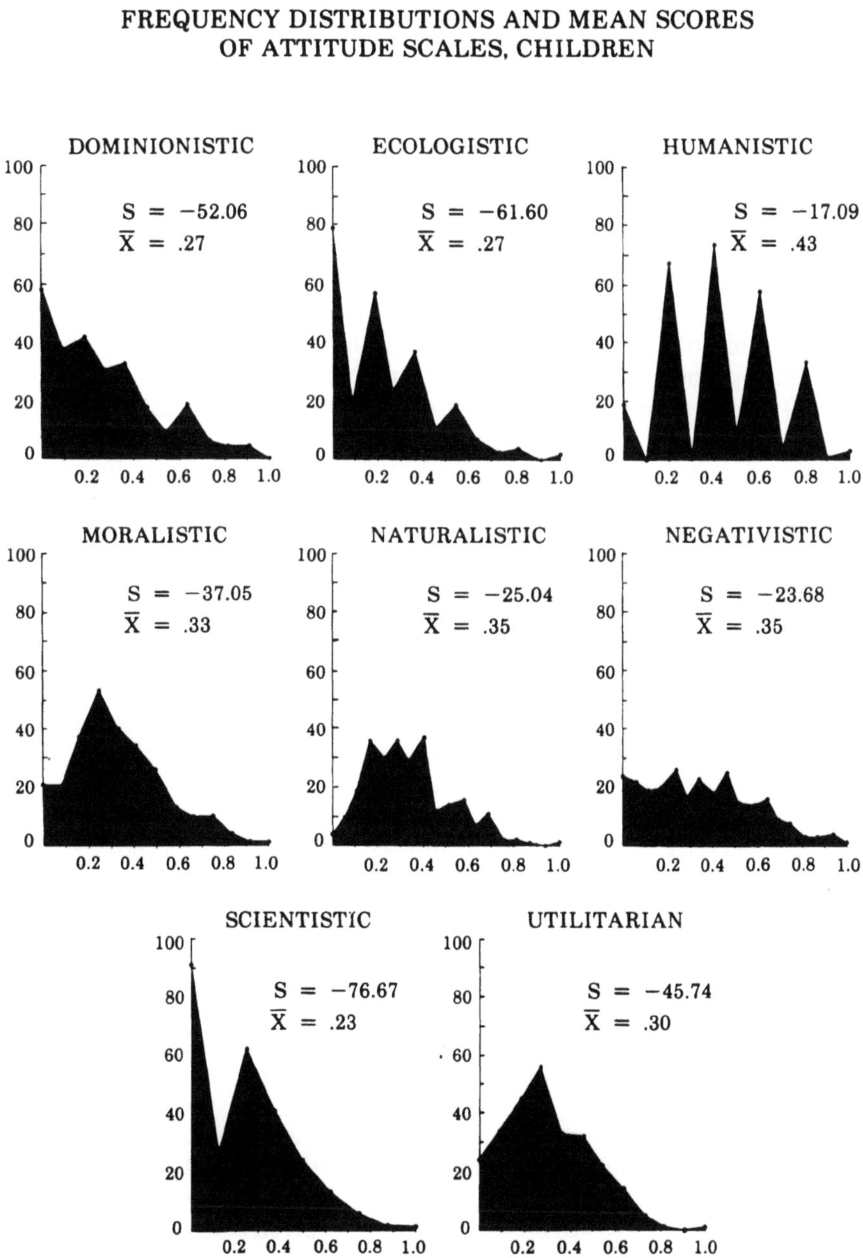

Vertical Axis: No. of Children Horizontal Axis: Standardized Mean Score

Table 4. Type of animal liked the most by all children

Beautiful animals	11.7%
Useful animals	8.8%
Animals that scientists study	5.6%
Loveable animals	38.8%
Animals in sports	9.1%
Animals in the woods	22.8%
Animals that are important to the balance of nature	4.2%

preferred type of animal, cited by 23% of the children.

The moralistic attitude ranked fourth in overall frequency of occurrence. Concern for the ethical treatment of animals was indicated by 70% of the children objecting to harvesting wild animals for their fur. Additionally, only 26% of the children supported hunting for recreational or sporting purposes, and 91% objected to trophy hunting, although 60% approved of hunting for food.

The utilitarian attitude was fifth in relative "popularity." By comparison, the greater frequency of the humanistic and naturalistic attitudes suggested children appreciate animals more for recreational and emotional than for practical reasons. Only 9% of the children cited "useful" animals as their favorite type of animal.

The dominionistic attitude was relatively uncommon, ranking sixth in frequency of occurrence. The least requently occurring attitudes were the ecologistic and scientistic. These latter attitudes emphasize an intellectual perspective of animals, suggesting that conceptual understandings of animals are somewhat uncommon among children. The rarity of the scientistic and ecologistic attitudes was also reflected in "scientifically interesting animals" being cited by 6%, and animals "important to the balance of nature" by 4%, of the children as their favorite types of animals.

In the national study of adults, the humanistic attitude was also the most frequent perspective of animals, and the negativistic and moralistic attitudes were similarly popular (Table 5). The most striking difference in attitudes towards animals between children and adults was the widely varying occurrence of the naturalistic and utilitarian perspectives. The naturalistic attitude was much more common among children, while a utilitarian view of animals was far more typical of adults.

Some impressive attitude differences occurred among children distinguished by age, sex, ethnicity, and urban/rural residence.

Significant age differences were observed on every scale with the

Table 5. National sample—18 years and older; childrens sample—2nd, 5th, 8th, 11th grades by attitude scale mean scores, slope of scale frequency distribution, and rank of occurence

	Adults			Children		
	$\overline{X}$	Slope based on actual response ranges	Rank of occurence	$\overline{X}$	Slope based on actual response ranges	Rank of occurence
Dominionistic	.14	− 746.08	7	.27	−52.06	5
Ecologistic	.22	− 603.25	5	.27	−61.60	5
Humanistic	.36	− 359.86	1	.43	−17.09	1
Moralistic	.27	− 375.90	3	.33	−37.05	4
Naturalistic	.20	− 578.32	6	.35	−25.04	2
Negativistic	.28	− 456.61	2	.35	−23.68	2
Scientistic	.10	−1143.45	8	.23	−76.67	8
Utilitarian	.23	− 398.21	4	.30	−45.74	4

exception of the humanistic (Table 6). Younger children consistently placed the needs of people over animals, and expressed minimal concern for the rights and protection of animals. This difference was reflected in highly significant utilitarian, dominionistic, and moralistic scale results. Younger children also expressed far less interest in animals, particularly wildlife. This difference was reflected in highly significant negativistic and naturalistic results. Finally, younger children were substantially less knowledgeable and informed about animals and the natural environment, as suggested by striking knowledge and ecologistic scale findings.

These results were somewhat surprising, perhaps due to our society's idealization of young children's perceptions of animals. The tendency is to believe young children have some natural affinity for living creatures, regarding them as little friends or kindred spirits. The results suggest otherwise, since young children were the most exploitative, unfeeling, and uninformed of all children in their attitudes toward animals. Some have argued our society creates a "make-believe" world for young children, often ill-preparing them for reality, and a related tendency may be a distortion of the actual views of young people toward animals. These results suggest educational efforts among children 6 to 10 years of age might best focus on the affective realm, mainly emphasizing emotional concern and sympathy for animals.

The most profound shift between 5th and 8th grade was a major

Table 6. Analysis of variance and multiple classification analysis results for grade by attitude and knowledge scales

	Sig F	$\overline{X}$ score	Devia. from mean after adj. for ind. & cov. variables		Sig F	$\overline{X}$ score	Devia. from mean after adj. for ind. & cov. variables
Dominionistic	.00			**Negativistic**	.00		
2nd grade		4.65	1.71			8.79	2.87
5th grade		3.26	0.24			6.29	0.12
8th grade		1.96	−1.35			5.12	− 0.87
11th grade		2.12	−0.56			4.04	− 1.98
Ecologistic	.00			**Scientistic**	.00		
2nd grade		2.00	−1.06			3.11	1.22
5th grade		2.43	−0.57			1.93	0.17
8th grade		3.03	0.26			1.06	− 0.87
11th grade		4.28	1.30			1.38	− 0.48
Humanistic	.67			**Utilitarian**	.00		
2nd grade		4.37	0.16			4.20	0.86
5th grade		4.26	−0.02			3.10	− 0.16
8th grade		3.45	−0.36			3.06	− 0.24
11th grade		4.52	−0.03			2.77	− 0.43
Moralistic	.01						
2nd grade		3.59	− 0.30				
5th grade		3.79	− 0.12				
8th grade		3.45	− 0.36				
11th grade		4.71	0.74				
Naturalistic	.01			**Knowledge**	.00		
2nd grade		5.89	0.03			30.50	−13.99
5th grade		5.53	−0.20			39.65	− 5.64
8th grade		5.18	−0.83			51.18	7.45
11th grade		6.84	0.97			55.11	11.57

The ages of children in the 2nd, 5th, 8th and 11th grades are (approximately): 6–7, 10, 13, and 16–18 years, respectively.

increase in factual knowledge of animals. The apparent value of emphasizing factual learning at this age is consistent with results reported by Horvat (1974), Dyar (1975), La Hart (1978), and Giles (1959).

Eleventh graders were far more ecologistic, moralistic, and naturalistic in their attitudes toward animals than were 8th graders. Activity results also suggested 11th grade children were far more interested in direct contact and recreational enjoyment of wildlife and the out-of-doors. The most basic change at this stage, thus, involved major increases in ethical concern for animals, appreciation of wildlife, and an ability to deal with abstract concepts such as ecosystems and biological diversity. This period appears to offer the best opportunity for developing ethical concern for animals and an understanding of ecology.

In summary, three major transitions were suggested by the results. The period from 2nd to 5th grade was most significantly characterized by a major increase in emotional concern and affection for animals. The years between 5th and 8th grades witnessed a dramatic improvement in factual and cognitive understanding of animals. Finally, the change from 8th to 11th grade was marked most of all by a major expansion in ethical and ecological concern for animals and the natural environment.

Highly significant differences among male and female children occurred on the dominionistic, ecologistic, humanistic, negativistic, and knowledge scales (Table 7). Moderately significant utilitarian scale results were also found. These results indicated greater factual knowledge, awareness and concern for wildlife among male children. On the other hand, female children were more inclined to oppose subordination and dominance of animals, and evidenced a greater emotional affection for large, attractive, primarily domestic pet animals.

Male/female differences on the humanistic, dominionistic and negativistic scales were significant at all age levels. Gender differences on

Table 7. Analysis of variance and multiple classification analysis results for sex by attitude and knowledge scales

	Sig F	$\overline{X}$ score	Devia. from mean after adj. for ind. & cov. variables		Sig F	$\overline{X}$ score	Devia. from mean after adj. for ind. & cov. variables
Dominionistic	.00			**Negativistic**	.00		
Male		3.61	0.64			5.18	−0.88
Female		2.34	−0.62			6.80	0.85
Ecologistic	.01			**Scientistic**	.89		
Male		3.36	0.39			1.83	−0.03
Female		2.60	−0.38			1.86	0.03
Humanistic	.01			**Utilitarian**	.09		
Male		3.93	−0.35			3.50	0.19
Female		4.65	0.34			3.06	−0.19
Moralistic	.27						
Male		3.73	−0.16				
Female		4.05	0.16				
Naturalistic	.66			**Knowledge**	.02		
Male		5.78	−0.13			47.03	2.47
Female		5.95	0.13			41.82	−2.39

the knowledge, ecologistic and moralistic scales, however, were inconsequential among 2nd grade children, although significant at all other age levels. An increase in moralistic concern among female students from 8th to 11th grades was particularly impressive. Male children, in contrast, became far more knowledgeable and concerned about wildlife and the natural environment than female children as they grew older.

Ethnic variations were striking on all the attitude scales with the exception of the moralistic and scientistic (Table 8). Far greater knowledge of animals and the natural enviroment among white children was particularly evident. Moreover, knowledge variations were as great in 2nd as 11th grade. Black children also expressed a greater willingness to subordinate animals, especially in the context of improving human material well-being. These differences were reflected in significant dominionistic and utilitarian scale results. Finally, black children revealed less affection and general interest in animals, particularly wildlife, as suggested by significant humanistic, negativistic, and naturalistic results.

Surprisingly few significant urban/rural differences were observed,

Table 8. Analysis of variance and multiple classification analysis results for ethnicity by attitude and knowledge scale

	Sig F	$\bar{X}$ score	Devia. from mean after adj. for ind. & cov. variables		Sig F	$\bar{X}$ score	Devia. from mean after adj. for ind. & cov. variables
Dominionistic	.01			**Negativistic**	.00		
White		2.74	−0.25			5.58	−0.16
Nonwhite		3.83	1.21			7.60	0.79
Ecologistic	.01			**Scientistic**	.18		
White		3.18	0.13			1.80	−0.08
Nonwhite		2.12	−0.66			2.19	0.39
Humanistic	.02			**Utilitarian**	.01		
White		4.41	0.19			3.13	−0.16
Nonwhite		3.50	−0.94			4.02	0.78
Moralistic	.39						
White		3.91	0.03				
Nonwhite		3.55	−0.14				
Naturalistic	.07			**Knowledge**	.00		
White		6.01	0.05			47.40	1.17
Nonwhite		5.05	−0.22			31.60	−5.72

with the exception of negativistic and knowledge scale results (Table 9). Rural children were more interested and knowledgeable about animals, particularly in contrast to children living in the large cities. Few major changes occurred among residential groups when controlling for age. One exception was a marked increase in knowledge of animals among suburban children.

Table 9. Analysis of variance and multiple classification analysis results for population present residence by attitude and knowledge scales

	Sig F	$\bar{X}$ score	Devia. from mean after adj. for ind. & cov. variables		Sig F	$\bar{X}$ score	Devia. from mean after adj. for ind. & cov. variables
Dominionistic	.24			**Negativistic**	.04		
Urban		3.04	−0.48			6.75	0.61
Small city		3.34	1.15			5.85	0.41
Suburb		3.19	−0.12			6.29	−0.32
Rural		2.42	−0.15			4.91	−0.68
Ecologistic	.38			**Scientistic**	.23		
Urban		2.71	−0.10			1.78	0.33
Small city		2.77	−0.53			1.45	−0.13
Suburb		3.11	0.42			2.06	−0.05
Rural		3.35	0.10			2.03	−0.15
Humanistic	.84			**Utilitarian**	.69		
Urban		4.15	0.18			3.39	−0.12
Small city		4.49	−0.01			3.15	0.20
Suburb		4.42	−0.04			3.44	0.03
Rural		4.30	−0.15			3.06	−0.04
Moralistic	.43						
Urban		3.92	−0.08				
Small city		4.23	0.30				
Suburb		4.02	0.31				
Rural		3.50	−0.40				
Naturalistic	.16			**Knowledge**	.00		
Urban		5.47	−0.49			38.00	−5.96
Small city		5.72	−0.09			46.90	−1.13
Suburb		5.79	−0.06			42.90	2.52
Rural		6.61	0.67			52.30	5.23

Attitude differences observed across all the demographic groups additionally revealed some interesting results, although these will be only briefly examined. On the negativistic scale, the highest scores were found among 2nd graders, nonwhites, female and urban children, in contrast to the low scores of 8th and 11th grade, rural resident, and male children (Figure 2). Ecologistic scores were highest among older children, male, and rural residents, in comparison to the low scores of 2nd graders and nonwhites (Figure 3). On the utilitarian scale, 2nd

Figure 2: Negativistic scale mean scores by children demographic groups

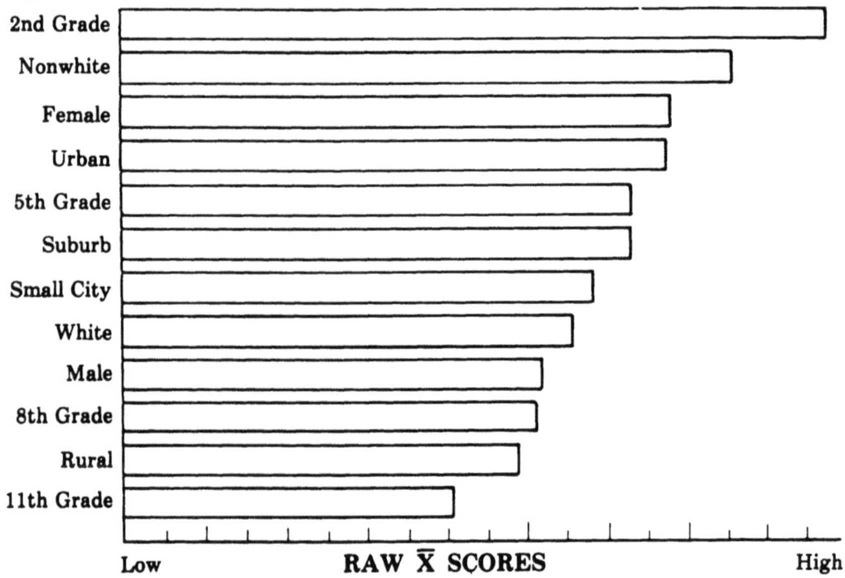

Figure 3: Ecologistic scale mean scores by children demographic groups

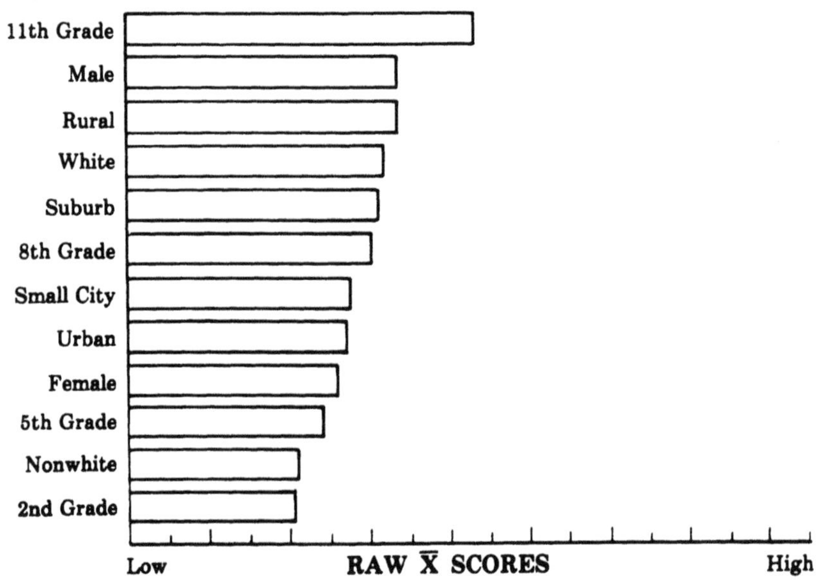

graders and nonwhites had the highest scores, while the lowest utilitarian scores occurred among 11th graders and female children (Figure 4).

Figure 4: Utilitarian scale mean scores by children demographic groups

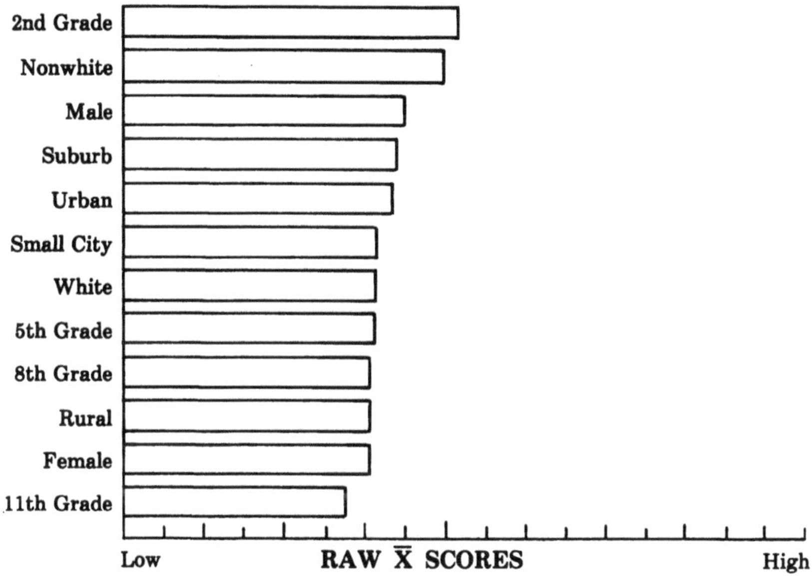

ACTIVITIES

The extent and influence of various activities involving animals will be briefly reviewed. Three-quarters or more of the children participated in seven animal-related activities during the previous two-year period including visiting zoos (93%), owning a pet (87%), fishing (87%), learning about animals in schools (83%), feeding birds (82%), reading books or magazines about animals (76%), and watching "Wild Kingdom" on television (74%). On the other hand, the least frequent activities included family livestock raising (21%), hunting (18%), trapping (13%), and belonging to an animal-related club (8%).

The attitude and knowledge scores of children who *frequently* participated in some of these activities were examined. Particularly surprising was the relatively low knowledge scores of children who learned about animals in school or who visited zoos (Table 10). Moreover, these two groups had the highest negativistic scale scores (Table 11). These activities, thus, appeared to exert little positive influence on children. Most zoological parks continue to fail to go beyond superficial entertainment toward instilling greater appreciation of animals among children, while most learning about animals in school appears to be so di-

Table 10. Knowledge scale mean scores by selected animal activity groups*

	Mean score
Ever hunted	51.77
Belong to animal club	51.23
Family raised livestock	47.09
Went outside to look at birds	45.85
Have a pet	45.63
Learned about animals in school	44.99
Went to zoo	44.89

*Most of these groups include only children who frequently participated in these activities. Significance tests were not performed because the groups were not mutually exclusive.

Table 11. Negativistic scale mean scores by selected animal activity groups

	Mean score
Went to zoo	5.94
Learned about animals in school	5.92
Went outside to look at birds	5.88
Ever fished	5.75
Family raised livestock	5.65
Have a pet	5.46
Belong to animal club	5.18
Ever hunted	3.89

vorced from direct experience with animals and the natural environment that little basic knowledge results.

More encouraging activity results were found among children who birdwatched, belonged to animal-related clubs, or hunted. These children were generally more appreciative, knowledgeable, and concerned about animals. These results suggest the positive value of direct, participatory contact between children and animals.

CONCLUSION

Perhaps the most outstanding result of this exploratory study was the indication of varying stages in the evolution of children's perceptions of animals. Each period appears to offer varying opportunities for environmental education. The transition from 2nd to 5th grade would seem the most opportune time for emphasizing affective/emotional concern for animals. The interval between 5th and 8th grades, on the other hand, offers the most promising possibilities for developing cognitive and factual understanding of animals. Finally, the shift from 8th to 11th grades would appear to be the most appropriate period for fostering ethical and ecological appreciation of animals and the natural world.

Ethnic and urban/rural findings suggest the need for devoting more attention to the animal-related perceptions and interests of urban disadvantaged children. Activity results indicate the value of educational programs that emphasize direct contact and experimental involvement with animals.

The results of this exploratory study clearly suggest the importance of more extensive and in-depth investigation of children's perceptions and relationships to animals. The reported findings intimate the possibility of exercising meaningful influence on the development of a more positive, informed, and benign perspective on animals among children. More ambitious and imaginative efforts will be required, however, as the eventual well-being of animals and the natural world will depend on the future commitment and concern of today's youth.

REFERENCES

Dyar, N.A. 1975. *Assessing environmental attitudes and behaviors of a seventh grade population.* Ph.D. dissertation. Berkeley: University of California.

Giles, R.H. Jr. 1959. *The conservation knowledge of Virginia school pupils.* Transactions North American Wildlife Natural Resource Conference, 29:488-97.

Horvat, R.E. 1974. *Fifth and eighth grade student orientation toward the environment and environmental problems.* Ph.D. dissertation, University of Wisconsin.

Kellert, S.R. 1979. *Public attitudes toward critical wildlife issues.* Order from U.S. Government Printing Office, Number 024-020-00-623-4, Washington, D.C.

Kellert, S.R. 1980a. *Activities of the American public relating to animals.* Order from U.S. Government Printing Office, Number 024-010-00-624-2, Washington, D.C.

Kellert, S.R. 1980b. Contemporary values of wildlife in American society. In: Shaw, W.W. and Zube, E.H. eds. *Wildlife Values.* Center for Assessment of Noncommodity Natural Resource Values, Institutional Series Report Number 1. U.S.D.A., Rocky Mountain Forest and Range Experiment Station, Fort Collins, Colorado, pages 31-60.

Kellert, S.R. and Berry, J.K. 1981. *Knowledge, affection and basic attitudes towards animals in American society.* Order from U.S Government Printing Office, Number 024-010-00-625-1, Washington, D.C.

Kellert, S.R. and Westervelt, M.O. 1982. *Trends in animal use and perceptions in 20th century America.* Order from U.S. Government Printing Office, Number 024-020-006-21-8, Washington, D.C.

LaHart, D.E. 1978. *The influence of knowledge on young people's perceptions about wildlife.* Final report to National Wildlife Federation, Washington, D.C.

Pomerantz, G.A. 1977. *Young peoples attitudes toward wildlife.* Division report number 2781, Michigan Department Natural Resources.

EMPATHY, HUMANENESS AND ANIMAL WELFARE

M. W. Fox

2100 L Street, N.W.
Washington, D.C. 20037

Empathy is defined variously as: the intellectual identification with or vicarious experiencing of the feelings, thoughts, or attitudes of another (*Random House Dictionary*); the power of projecting one's personality into and so fully understanding the object of contemplation (*Oxford Dictionary*); and the imaginative projection of one's own consciousness into another being (*Webster's Dictionary*).

Sympathy and empathy are distinctly different phenomena. Sympathy is the sharing of another's emotions, especially grief and anguish, involving pity and compassion. Empathy (from the Greek term meaning affection, and a more recent German term *einfuhlung*, which means "a feeling in"), entails the power of *understanding* and imaginatively entering into another's feelings. While the two are not mutually exclusive, empathy implies some level of objective knowledge and therefore a greater accuracy of perception and affect than are seen in sympathy, which, because it is more subjective, may be a less accurate and more intuitive way of perceiving and responding to another's emotions. In our relations with animals (as with each other), sympathetic concern may or may not be misplaced, while empathetic concern, since it includes both objective understanding (of both the animal's nature and our ethical responsibilities) and emotional involvement, is likely to be more accurate and, therefore, less often confounded by anthropomorphic projections.

Empathy is motivated by *concern*, the accuracy of that concern (a desert animal doesn't need water even if one is thirsty observing it in the Sahara) being a condition of *understanding*: of rational objective ("scientific") knowledge. From right understanding, right action, a compassion (and responsible stewardship) arises. The sympathetic experiences, feelings, and imaginings (of how one might feel in the other's place) that come from empathizing (i.e., the introjections of one's projections) become more accurate with experience and rational understanding. This is the key to good human relations and the humane treatment of animals.

In relation to a person's emotional rapport with an animal, is empathy possible? Sympathetic concern for animals is often judged, sometimes correctly, as being a sentimental, anthropomorphic projection. Sheer subjective sympathy toward an animal, without objective understanding of its behavior and needs, can lead to erroneous assumptions as to its well-being, and to misjudgement of others' treatment of animals as being cruel. Empathy is possible when the "feelings, thoughts, or attitudes of another" can be vicariously experienced: thus when there is objective knowledge about what an animal's overt behavior signifies, and what emotional states, intentions, and expectations such overt behavior reflects, empathy *is* possible. Without such objective knowledge, we have sympathy and varying degrees of anthropomorphization. Understanding and sympathy combined make empathy possible.

Empathy is a perceptual and cognitive phenomenon, not simply an anthropomorphic "humanizing" projection: it is analogous to what phenomenologist Merleau-Ponty terms lateral coexistential knowledge as distinct from objective, "vertical" (i.e., Cartesian mind over body) knowing and perceiving. Dallery (1978) illustrates this mode of perception as follows:

> *This is not the place to summarize Merleau-Ponty's magisterial work,* The Phenomenology of Perception *(1946). For our purposes, it is important to note that perception is described as the complex, always open, temporal "access" between world and perceiver. It is neither a causal process nor a process distinct from social relations, speech, or understanding (as it would be if perception were a "thought of seeing"). So in perceiving a snake, for example, I do not simply receive an impression of a sinuous form having a certain mottled pattern; I do not see a cold, indifferent fact, or have a bunch of impressions to which I might or might not endow some value depending on my feelings; I see the* snake, *which is to say that I see its behavior in an environment proper to it and that I "appropriate" the snake's way of being, the snake's perception of certain things around it. But I am free to regard the snake as an object and admire its beauty, or to loathe its slithering.*

There is knowledge and feeling inherent in such empathetic perception. Dallery continues:

> *To see the animal moving in its environment is already to "care" about the animal, since in a way I put myself in its place. I say it is foraging, or mating, or fleeing; I know what it is doing because these are analogues of my behavior...But if beasts have no interior being and are automata, as Descartes held, I cannot "think in their place." In fact, I cannot really perceive them. They become real to me only as I add to certain sensations meanings that come from my sentiment of intellect. In outline, this is the tendency of modern thought. Perception is relegated either to blind mechanisms (as in skeptical empiricism and objective psychology) or to operations of the mind (as in Cartesianism and Kantianism). For Husserl and Merleau-Ponty, this amounts to canceling out perception and losing the world (at least losing it in and by means of philosophy). Merleau-Ponty then is not speaking metaphorically when he charges both camps in the modern tradition with blindness; he does not mean blindness to things in the environment (loss of the ability to see) but blindness to the world as lived, the world as open to environments of other beasts, as providing the ground of our coexistence of being together.*

This I call simply a lack of empathy, which makes us dehumanize ourselves by objectifying the world, the causes of which need careful study.

From the existential phenomenologist's perspective, the difference between detached objectivity and rational empathy can be viewed as follows. Dallery (1978) equates the former with "vertical" Cartesian, hierarchical, instrumental, perceptional knowledge and the latter with "lateral" coexistential knowledge and perception. So where does sympathy fit into this paradigm? Dallery does not answer this question. It lies, I believe, in the "lateral" or coexistential dimension as the potential bridge for rational empathy and coexistential knowledge. And it is easily inhibited by the "vertical" dimension of Cartesian thought and perception. Hence Cartesianism, while not inhibiting rational intellectual development, can impair the expression of sympathy which is a prerequisite for the development of rational empathy and moral maturity.

The Cartesian dimension is advantageous to our survival or being and the coexistential dimension vital for our becoming. In thinking and perceiving in both these objective and trans-subjective dimensions, we literally think and see both ways, a "double-vision" that reconciles the dialectical nature of reality and the duality of self and other, with the paradoxical wisdom of objective love. Then, and only then, is a mature, rationally responsible and empathetic love and understanding of others possible. Both meaning and fulfillment are then experienced as a kind of resonance between love and understanding: *agapé* and *logos*.

There are those who believe that since the subjective world of animals cannot be objectively weighed and measured, it does not exist. Furthermore, empathizing seems pointless since animals do not really have emotions or an inner subjective mental world, except one governed by unconscious instincts. This animal-as-machine attitude, termed Cartesianism after the philosopher René Descartes who gave this attitude scientific respectability in the seventeenth century, is not the only factor that impairs our ability to empathize.

The ability to empathize may be inborn as an adaptive component of our sociobiology, and as Alice Miller (1981) has shown, lack of mature parental love and understanding can severely impair a child's empathetic development.

The experience of parents' empathetic understanding (expressed as the ability to deal supportively with the child's suffering, anxieties, and growing independence) has a significant influence upon a child's ability to love and empathize. Males, in our patriarchal society, may well show more cruelty toward animals, or justify the same, because they close off empathy more than females when faced with others' helplessness and suffering. The more intense, existential anxiety and reduced ability to empathize, plus a greater need to assume dominion over others (as power and control) in the male of our species may be rooted in the male child's greater sense of insecurity and separateness from the mother in early life. This is less intense in little girls because they have the security and connectedness of maternal gender identity. Hence women may be better able to empathize and cope with others' suffering, this sex difference being exemplified by the greater nurturing ability of females that may be more than a culturally determined sex-stereotype. The greater the sense of personal security, the less need for such distancing defense mechanisms to cope with anxiety as rationalization, denial, sublimation, objectification and reaction formation.

Those adult males who are less "feminine," empathetic and nurturing, are not necessarily less sensitive than women. Their apparent insensitivity may be attributed to an emotional closing down to varying degrees when faced with others' helplessness and suffering. This awakens their own unbearable feelings of vulnerability, fear of being hurt and of losing control or of being controlled. Fear and empathy are thus linked, when empathizing evokes the awareness and terror of one's own ultimate non-being. The fears of empathy's burdens and of losing power and control are the greatest obstacles to man's being and becoming humane. To judge such people as being deliberately cruel or intrinsically insensitive is surely unjust, yet this is a common reaction in the humane, animal welfare and rights movement.

Such defensive ideologies as patriarchal dominionism and Cartesianism, like machismo, are perhaps reaction formations in the service of the ego, especially of the insecure male ego, in this culture, which need to be recognized as pathologically maladaptive reaction formations.

The ability to empathize is also affected by cultural attitudes and values: emotions are put down by instrumental rationalists as being irrational and subjective. Self-serving religious and political ideologies also impair the ability to empathize, notably such ideologies as: man's God-given dominion (over women, animals and nature); of God being only transcendent and not also ominpresent, inhering in all living things. Beliefs that animals have an intrinsic right to exist, or are ensouled, or possess a spark of inherent divinity, have been dismissed as "eastern" philosophy and pagan pantheism. Yet respect and compassion toward all of God's creations is an integral part of Christianity (especially of Paulist, Gnostic and Essene doctrines).

The moral foundation of our industrial civilization's relationship with animals and nature is clearly flawed by its lack of reverence for all life. In order to further the exploitation of animals by the biomedical, farming and wildlife "resource" industries, such beliefs in man's dominion and in animals having no inherent rights, divinity or capacity to suffer emotionally, become essential defenses to rationalize away and deny empathetic feelings of compassion, guilt and responsibility.

There are a number of other reasons why empathy toward animals is impaired, leading to their being treated inhumanely or with indifference. First, we lack objective, scientific knowledge, (rather than applied production-related information) about the behavioral requirements and emotional, subjective world of animals. Farmers, animal scientists and others involved in livestock production also have little or no formal training in ethology. A stockman who knows his animals, who can "think like a pig," for example, usually does a better job than one that lacks this basic and essential knowledge.

Second, desensitization, a blunting of sensitivity, occurs naturally as a defense mechanism when one has to perform various painful procedures upon animals and must ultimately kill them or send them to slaughter. Empathy is thus withdrawn, because the burden of responsible compassion that comes with empathizing with another's suffering and helplessness awakens one's own sense of vulnerability and death awareness, which can be unbearable. Many people seem to confuse empathy with being anthropomorphic probably because they are repressing their own true feelings behind a defensive screen of intellectual rationalizations used to justify and protect vested interests in animal exploitation and to alleviate feelings of guilt. Closing off empathy, especially in laboratory animal research (with its scientific "objectivity") and factory farming and wildlife exploitation (with their objectification of animals as "stock," "food converters," "resources," and "trophies,") ultimately distorts perceptions and objectivity, and becomes a primary source of needless animal abuse and suffering.

Third, the empathetic burden of responsibility is lightened further by making economic and other rationalizations to justify certain procedures: i.e., that suffering is necessary, unavoidable, and justifiable if any societal benefits are accrued.

What may be termed "protective objectification"—the denial of others' subjectivity—in order to avoid closeness, responsibility, and the burdens of empathy, is another obstacle, exemplified by women being treated as "sex objects," medical patients as "cases," and animals as trophies, pets, research tools, livestock, etc. Many persons in a paradoxical and potentially stressful relationship will often mobilize the above defenses since emotional involvement can lead euphemistically to "burn-out": farmers who nurture animals that will be killed; animal shelter personnel who are concerned about animal welfare but must euthanize them; biomedical researchers and laboratory technicians who care for animals but cause them to suffer and mutilate, kill and dissect them; physicians and nurses attending the terminally ill, knowing they will soon die. While such persons must be "realists" in dealing with the paradoxes of life, the difference between a nurturing and supportive person and one who is empathetically disconnected is the difference between humaneness and indifference, between compassion and inhumanity. The difference is not between intrinsically kind and cruel persons, but between those who can bear the burden of empathy and those who fear it. The difference between a humane farm and a large "factory" farm, and regular human hospital and a hospice for the dying is surely based upon the individual's capacity to empathize and to not protectively shut out the realities of life's suffering and the finality of one's own non-being.

Protective objectification is analogous to Judaic philosopher Martin Buber's "I-It" relationship. From Buber's perspective (1970), empathy enables us to break out of the objective, detached "I-It" mind-set into the trans-subjectively objective realm of "I-Thou." The objective and subjective realms of each "It" and "Thou" are mutually inclusive: every entity is a dualistic monad. The subjective, intrinsic value or worth of one entity is part of the objective, instrumental realm of other interdependent monads (be they atoms or living beings), that are bound in relationship (which may be purely physical, ecological, social or emotional). In Buber's terms, the subjective "I" of one monadic entity is the objective "It" of another. But when there is respect for the "I-ness" or subjective realm of another's being, and empathetic love and compassionate understanding, the objective "It" becomes another subjectively resonant, spiritual "Thou." A monadic relationship is then made, through respect and love, which is, for Man, the emotional, spiritual and ethical manifestation and experience of a unified field of being. This state of relatedness does not, I believe, as Buber suggests, exclude or transcend the "I-It" objective duality, but rather enfolds it in love, such that the objective instrumental realm is still an intrinsic part of the relationship but does not govern it.

Buber's concept of "I-Thou" embodies the spiritual and political principles of reverence for all life, humane stewardship, respect, nurturance, "reciprocal maintenance," co-evolution and agapé (as self-giving love). Objective instrumental rationalism and love are not mutually exclusive, but rather they reconcile, at the conscious, ethical level of reality, the dialectical, paradoxical antinomies of life. The exclusion of love from objectivity brings evil and suffering into the world, which cause increasing anxiety, which in turn leads to more power and control over others or emotional withdrawal, and to more evil and suffering.

The "otherness" of an animal Buber (1970) describes eloquently when he strokes a horse at his grandparents' estate:

> *I must say that what I experienced in touch with the animal was the Other, the immense otherness of the Other, which, however, did not remain strange like the otherness of the ox and the ram, but rather let me draw near and touch it...and yet it let me approach, confided itself to me, placed itself elementally in the relation of Thou and Thou with me.*

Buber emphasizes that an "I-Thou" rather than an "I-It" relationship is therefore possible in the absence of a reciprocal observing ego, as when one contemplates a rock, or nature, or interacts with an animal. It is possible in such moments of openness with the nonhuman world to actualize and encounter the spiritual essence of Being that inheres in all animate and inanimate forms and for Man, therefore, to discover, if not actually bestow meaning and significance, not as objective knowledge or some projected ideology of animism or panpsychism but as a panentheistic gnosis of the divinity or spiritual quality within all: an expanding state of pan-relation with the *anima mundi*, soul of the Earth, or God within.

Buber writes that the unity and living wholeness of a tree is manifest to those who say "Thou" and is present when *they* are present. It is they who grant the tree the opportunity to manifest its being, but most often our habitual attitudes, ways of thinking, perceiving and relating, deny us such a relationship. In Buber's words:

> *Spirit become word, spirit become form—whoever has been touched by the spirit and did not close himself off knows to some extent of the fundamental fact: neither germinates and grows in the human world without having been sown; both issue from encounters with the other.*

That most animals are capable of experiencing and expressing affection and of enjoying life in their way, as we do in ours, and like us have interests, means that they are emotionally and cognitively, and some would say spiritually, little different from us. That we are different in terms of our power of dominion over them does not mean that we can ignore the ethical relevance of these similarities. We differ in degree and not in kind: we are not superior, but our objectifying of the world leads us to believe so as we no longer perceive the unified field of all Being.

Comparative sciences such as zoology, ethology, physiology, and psychology, reveal how sapience and sentience—intelligence and conscious sensitivity—evolve. The only differences between humans and other animals, which create no discontinuity but build upon the phylogenetic and ontogenetic sequence, are our powers of self-contemplation, creative imagination and verbal conceptualization and communication. The two axes of sapience and sentience reach their highest expression phylogenetically and ontogenetically in humans, as understanding and compassion, as the will is consciously motivated by the subjective force of love and directed by the objective power of knowledge. Knowledge applied without love is as self-serving, self-limiting and destructive as the love of narcissism's ignorance. Empathy, the synthesis of concern and sympathetic understanding of others, a quality not lacking in other animals, is the very essence of humane being.

CONCLUSION: HUMANENESS AS LOVE

Neither legislation nor moral codes can make people empathize with animals. Being humane is an attitude of heart and mind, of empathy and understanding, not simply a legal or moral injuction. At best, laws and codes guide and constrain human actions, but they do not inspire the ability to "love thy neighbor (and fellow creatures) as thyself." The one strong point of animal rights philosophy is that it draws our attention to the animals' own wants, intrinsic worth and interests. This implies that we and they have something in common: a will, a life of one's own, perhaps a soul. This is speaking closer to the heart. Recognition of these qualities in other beings awakens the heart of humility and compassion, fundamental tenets of all religious teachings. Being humane thus entails the spiritual recognition and affirmation, through empathy, humility, and compassion, of the divinity and sanctity of Self within all beings, within one's own self as well as within others.

The Buddha proclaimed: "One thing only do I teach: suffering and cease of suffering. Kindness to all living creatures is the true religion."

Likewise Pantanjali (circa 300 B.C.) gave the first step in yogic (religious) discipline as "the avoidance of injury to all living creatures," because all creatures were regarded as being part of God's creation and therefore sacred and ensouled with a spark of the Divine.

Humaneness is an expression of mature love that resacralizes nature, and all living things, not animistically but panentheistically in accord with the Christian (Paulist, Gnostic and Essene) doctrines of a divine omnipresent (as well as transcendent) Creator within all of creation, which is the basis of Schweitzer's theosophy of reverence for all life.

Empathy is the bridge for unconditional love, a love synonymous with experiencing the world without the domination of personal interests and preconceptions. Such a mature love is therefore revelationary, since it is the perception of the miraculous, of the numinously radiant divinity in all. This is the subjective recognition of Self in other, and thus of self-realization.

Through empathy, mature love is possible: such love is nondialectical in its arbitrary, unconditional non-duality of the observer (the lover) and the object of one's contemplation (as I-Thou). And love is paradoxical, for instead of losing one's sense of individuality, the sense and meaning of self is enhanced. Love transcends the paradoxical dualities of the subject-object manifolds of our every day enculturated reality, consciousness, and unconscious ego defenses. Love is revolutionary, because through the bridge of empathy, understanding as coexistential knowledge, is possible. This is the beginning of self-realization; of personal and interpersonal development and human evolution.

Gilligan (1983) links empathy with moral maturity. When both intellect and empathy are integrated in our thinking, "it joins the heart and the eye in an ethic that ties the activity of thought to the activity of care." Without such an integration, purely intellectual, rational thinking is objectifying and potentially alienating, since it limits empathetic understanding. A purely sympathetic response is a subjective projection and potentially inappropriate, and no less damaging, than a purely objective response. Informed sympathy is empathy, expressed as compassionate understanding. Rational empathy is the only basis for ethically responsible behavior.

Insofar as the humane movement is concerned, and humane education in particular, to evoke sympathy for mistreated animals (for fund-raising purposes or to stimulate students' and supporters' moral indignation) is unethical if it is based only upon the sentiment of abolishing all suffering and not also upon respect for animals' intrinsic worth and recognition of the importance of humane ethics and reverence for all life to our moral development and social change.

We live in two worlds: the objective and the subjective. When we make the two worlds one, and put the inside on the outside, as Jesus once said, we will discover the Kingdom of Heaven, or in modern parlance, reality as a unified field of being. As animals, we live in our subjectivity, and as rational beings we stand apart from the world in our intellectually rational objectivity. In the one is kinship; in the other, power: but together we have the possibility of mature, responsible relationship and planetary stewardship. Apart, we have delusion, oppression, and destruction, creating the imbalances that we perceive as evil, and experience as suffering. By introducing empathy and using power and control over life in order to avoid the feelings of vulnerability and helplessness in the face of life's burdens of suffering and death, we cause even more suffering. The barrier between these two worlds, which Buber termed "I-It" and "I-Thou", is not our objectivity, or our subjectivity. Both are essential attributes of our being and becoming. But they must become integrated with the unified field of our own being that embraces animals and nature, for we are both. To perceive and think otherwise is to remain unintegrated, which is the ultimate barrier to our self-realization and moral maturity. We, animals and Nature are one. In order to change the world, we must first become as one with the world (in peace and harmony). And since peace comes from within, we must first see to ourselves before we can change the world. Then the way of empathy is clear.

POSTSCRIPT

Why Do Animal Shelters Kill So Many Pets?

Psychiatrist M. Scott Peck in *A Road Less Travelled* draws a very pertinent, which some would see as impertinent, correlation between the love people have for their pets and the high rate of divorce among G.I.'s who lost affection for their Viet Nam and Korean wives as they began to learn English, and assert their no longer dependent and subordinate individuality. Puppies and kittens likewise lose their appeal to many as they mature, assert their independence and individuality. And so like G.I. brides, they are abandoned because, beneath the complaints that they are disobedient, too much trouble, or have annoying habits and behavioral problems, they are no longer loved.

The mass destruction of some 13 million unwanted, abandoned, and neglected cats and dogs each year in the U.S. must assuredly reflect the limitations of an immature, narcissistic love relationship, an aspect of the human–companion animal bond which has been grossly neglected by researchers and is not simply a consequence of "unthinking and uneducated" owners. Peck defines mature love as "the will to extend one's self for the purpose of nurturing one's own and another's spiritual growth." In our relationships with captive and domesticated animals, this is surely the essence of humane husbandry. It is the absence of empathy, compassion and understanding, which undergirds all inhumane and unethical relations between people and between us and the animals, as they continue to be exploited for selfish, emotional, financial, and other reasons.

Farmers and biomedical researchers can put their empathy, compassion, and understanding of animals on one side for reasons of profit and instrumental utility, arguing that the extreme privations of factory farming and mental and physical suffering of laboratory cats, dogs, primates, and other animals, is for the "benefit of society." A society that can find anything of greater value than empathy, compassion, and wisdom is perhaps suffering from the pathology of materialism and objectivity. The divorced G.I.'s bride was simply the material of his narcissistic yearnings; a sexual object. Likewise cats and dogs can be status or play objects, or things to fondle or control; and farm animals simply biological machines in the computerized technology of agribusiness; and laboratory animals mere components of experimental design and ultimate execution.

Fortunately not all husbands (G.I.'s) and husbanders (pet owners, farmers, and biomedical researchers) relate to other living beings in this way. But unfortunately, we must surmise that they are a minority, for to date they have been relatively silent on matters concerning human and animal rights. Or are they the silent majority? It is surely time to break the silence, after reflecting upon the monetary value of animals, for as Jesus said: "Do not two sparrows sell for a coin of small value? Yet not one of them will fall to the ground without your Father's knowledge; not one of them goes forgotten before God." (*Matthew* 10:29; *Luke* 12:6).

It is too simplistic to say that people love their pets because pets are "nonthreatening others." Perhaps by understanding why so many people find it easy to love animals, we may discover ways to help people love each other, and not be afraid to love, and those who hate, fear, or are indifferent toward animals, love them also, as *significant*, rather than as nonthreatening, others.

If love is the union of souls, then the bridge is empathy when such non-sentimental love is based upon compassion, respect, and understanding. Such love entails an openness of feeling, a degree of vulnerability, intolerable in the presence of any human or animal that is perceived, correctly or incorrectly, as being threatening. Fear inhibits the ability to give and receive love. Likewise, others' expectations that we feel we must live up to, set up defenses and roles. But with animals (and little children) when we have no fear toward them, and they have no demanding expectations of us, then we are free to love them.

Mature love is also impaired when the object of one's perception and even claimed affection, is exploited to one's own selfish advantage. Such exploitation, be it of a spouse or an animal companion (as a "pet," or for its pelt, meat, or physiological responses to test drugs), objectifies the potential "Thou" of the others' being into an "it" (a sex object, a child-substitute, a financial or intellectual gain, etc.). These objectifying transformations may seem necessary for our well-being, and to a degree they are. But when we transgress ethical boundaries in relating to others exploitatively rather than with empathetic understanding and respect, we limit our own potential fulfillment from such a relationship. This fulfillment is to become human, or even, as Plato and Aristotle envisioned, to "become like divinity as much as that is within our power."

REFERENCES

Buber, M. 1970. *I and Thou*, Walter Kaufman transl. New York:Scribners.
Dallery, C. 1978. In:Fox, M.W. and Morris, R.K. eds. *On the fifth day: Animal rights and human ethics*. Washington, D.C.:Acropolis Press. pp. 70-92.
Gilligan, C. 1983. *In a different voice*. Boston: Harvard University Press.
Miller, A. 1981. *Prisoners of childhood*. New York:Basic Books.

HUMAN/ANIMAL COMMUNICATION: CETACEAN ROLES IN HUMAN THERAPEUTIC SITUATIONS

M. Patricia Hindley*

Department of Communication
Simon Fraser University
Burnaby, B.C.
Canada, V5A 1S6

INTRODUCTION

A review of the literature on the relationship between animal and human indicates that whales and dolphins may have a mutually beneficial role to play in human therapeutic situations. Florida researchers have discovered that interaction with dolphins has favourably altered the behaviour of neurologically impaired people, and of autistic children who are usually withdrawn and uncommunicative.

Explorations with both wild and captive cetaceans may find suggestive direction from extensive research currently being done with pets and domestic animals. Growing scientific evidence suggests that animals can benefit not only the physically and mentally ill, the lonely and the incarcerated, but also the minds and bodies of healthy people as well. Research done at, for example, the University of Pennsylvania's Center for Interaction of Animals and Society, the University of Minnesota's Center for Study of Human-Animal Relationships

*Paper presented at the IWC Non-Consumptive Utilization of Cetacean Resources Conference, Boston, June 1983.

and Environments, the University of Cambridge, and by members of the Society for Companion Animal Studies in Paris, indicates marked therapeutic benefits from the involvement of animals in a variety of human situations.

DOMESTIC ANIMALS

In healthy people it has been found that animals act as "social lubricants," that is, they facilitate social interactions between owners and other people which often result in friendships (Mugford and M'Comisky 1974; Messent 1982). They provide companionship, affection and tactile contact for people whether they live alone or not. It seems to be a reciprocal exchange of affection and contact between human and animal. People report greater feelings of self-esteem, of having permission to be overtly affectionate, and to openly touch and fondle (the latter reported especially by men). They also felt animals allowed them to forget themselves and their problems and to engage in playfulness.

Interestingly enough there is little evidence to suggest that more than a small minority of people use animals as a substitute for human companionship. Rather an animal is seen as an "addition to," albeit an important one (Adell-Bath et al., 1979). In one study done by Katcher (1981), about 80% of the participants regarded their animals "as a person" and talked to them regularly. The value of a companion who does not "talk back" or criticize, seems to be of particular importance in the early lives of children.

Boris Levinson, a pioneer in the field of animal/children bond research, has demonstrated the value of pet animals in child development (Levinson 1969, 1972, 1978). Pets, he claims, can be major sources of emotional support, acting as friend and confidante, providing a constant source of love and tactile affection. They also enable the child to learn how to take responsibility and care for another, they also can provide disciplinary models. During times of bereavement, loss or similar stress, children with animal companions often fare better—the animal seems to provide continuity.

Levinson has also written about the use of animals in psychotherapy with children. He identifies a pattern in which the child first talks only to the dog, ignoring the therapist, then includes the therapist in the conversations with the dog, thus eventually able to deal directly with the therapist. For disturbed and psychotic children an animal may be the only animate object with which they can make contact in their struggle to establish positive human relationships again (Searles 1960). The unquestioning loyalty, total acceptance and uninhibited affection of the animal seem to be key factors in successful therapy with children whose communication with adults has either ceased or become disturbed. Successful work has been done with physically handicapped children in West Germany. It was found, for instance, that pet horses were very popular. Seated high in the saddle, a wheelchair-bound child could for once in her life look down on everyone and "maintain a sense of dignity."

Animals have also been used successfully with adults in mental hospitals, especially with those patients for whom all "other available therapeutic methods failed to bring about significant improvement" (Corson, Corson, and Alexander 1980). The patients were withdrawn, uncommunicative, self-centered, almost mute and psychologically bedridden. The introduction of an animal saw a gradual but significant shift towards self-esteem, responsibility and independence with increased mobility and a reaching out to others.

Similar success has been achieved by the Corsons, using pets on geriatric wards. One elderly man who had not spoken for 26 years, spontaneously said "You brought that dog," upon receiving a dog as a long-shot part of therapy. He later made friends and became quite an accomplished painter of animals. The introduction of birds to geriatric wards and to elderly people living alone has had quite remarkable positive effects from raising self-esteem, creating group cohesion, making friends, to maintaining health (Mugford and M'Comisky 1974). The researchers commented on the "surprisingly intimate and presumably rewarding attachment to these unsolicited pet birds." The typical view of a geriatric ward population as helpless, hopeless, and waiting to die becomes quite the opposite as normal healthy responses to life dormant in the company of our own kind, are triggered by other species.

This has also been true at Lima State Hospital in Ohio, a maximum security institution housing about 400 patients, including psychopaths and sex offenders. To date nearly 100 patients are involved in pet facilitated therapy. The 85% attempted suicide rate in the hospital in general dropped to zero seven years ago on those wards involved in pet therapy, and has remained there. The hospital has 20 aquaria and 160 animals including parrots, gerbils, rabbits, hamsters, guinea pigs and deer. While controlled studies need to be done, positive indications are the giving of humane and loving care to animals and improved social relationships. Similar results have been obtained with the use of farm animals and pets in psychotherapy with delinquent children in residential schools (Levinson 1972). Again the emotional and tactile contact with loving, non-critical animals may help diffuse feelings of hostility, alienation and rejection common in criminal offenders and anti-social behaviour.

EXPERIMENTAL ANIMALS

Evidence indicates that benefits accruing to us from the animal/human bond are not only psychosocial but also physiological. It has been found that in healthy people blood pressure and pulse rate drops when, for example, petting or talking to their animals, or when viewing a tank of tropical fish. In contrast blood pressure and heart rate increase when talking to other people, reading aloud, but again can be reduced if an animal is present in the room (Katcher and Friedmann 1980). The same researchers also found that the ownership of a pet was the factor most highly correlated with one year survival following a heart attack, apart from the physiological severity of the disease. Exercise and need for companionship were rejected as the main explanations since the group of patients included both married and single people, and also owners of small house-bound pets. Rather it may be that "dumb as opposed to speaking companions" offer a fuller explanation since "the speechless kind of companionship shared with pets may provide a source of relaxation that human companions who demand talk as the price of companionship may not provide" (Friedmann et al., 1980).

For experimental work done with animals in the laboratory during which animals are often subjected to abhorrent levels of pain and deprivation, it has been found that similar benefits accrue to the animal if they are in the presence of a sympathetic human. This is even more true if they are in physical contact. Such benefits are reduction of anxiety, lowering of blood pressure and heart rate, and increase in coronary blood flow.

Twenty years ago Gantt conducted research on the "effect of person" or effect of human contact on animals. He found significant variations in heart rate when an electric shock was administered to a dog's foot when the animal was alone and when it was being petted by a person. While being petted the heart rate increase was reduced by half. Similarly when the dog received a warning bell signalling the approach of shock, heart rate increased dramatically. If a person petted the dog during both bell and shock then the increase in heart rate was either eliminated or even reduced (Gantt et al., 1966). Clearly, human contact had made an enormous difference lending some credence to Darwin's belief that petting and contact in animals was an expression of love. Such experimental findings suggest that the animal/human bond is as important to the animal as it is to the human.

Other laboratory findings indicate emotional reactions in animals which closely parallel human behaviour, making reciprocity in the relationship even more believable. While much behaviour is species specific and it is dangerous to generalize to human behaviour, nevertheless, the parallels throw valuable light on the nature of the human/animal bond. According to some researchers emotional disorders such as anorexia, depression, neurotic behaviour, perversions, and criminal disorders have been observed in farm animals and pets, all intelligible in terms of recent stress or early history (Saul 1962).

The classic work of Harlow and his colleagues on total deprivation of tactile companionship in infant monkeys indicates similar emotional reactions to stress. One of the most interesting findings was the constant selection of the cloth surrogate mother during times of anxiety and insecurity even though the wire surrogate mother provided milk. It seemed that contact comfort was of overwhelming importance. Experiments in which infant monkeys could see but not touch their mothers, produced similar but less intense disturbances and distress. A further unexpected finding was that even though the cloth mother was inanimate, the infant felt such emotional security through warmth and body contact alone, that it was able to explore new objects in its surroundings. It was once thought by Harlow that infant monkeys reared from birth to six months in total isolation would never exhibit normal behaviour. However more recently he reports that if the right kind of body contact is provided, the behaviour is reversible (Suomi, Harlow, and McKinney 1972).

For instance, artificially inseminated mothers reared in isolation sometimes succumb to the pestering to cling by their determined offspring, such that they rear their second born normally. Secondly, heated cloth surrogate mothers given to six month old isolates produces positive social behaviour after a few weeks of intense clinging. Similar results are achieved when normal but younger pre-aggressive infants are placed in cages with six month old isolates. While the isolate withdraws, the normal infant's tendency is to cling. Again body contact is influential with the isolate. Another interesting observation of animal need for contact was reported by Coelho (1980). He observed a baboon in a primate colony adopt a feral kitten. As in the case of the human/pet bond the baboon was seen to hold the kitten close, to pet it and to use it as a social facilitator in interactions with other baboons.

Findings therefore show that two main elements in the animal/human bond are trust and touch. In the case of humans as has been said, there is ample evidence that a warm trusting and trustworthy non-human creature is often a key to health. In the case of both animal and human, it seems clear from the data that the addition of touch has not only positive and emotional effect on both, but is essential for normal development. Montagu (1978) reminds us of the general embryological law which says that the earlier a sensory system becomes functional, the more fundamental it is likely to be. Since touch is the earliest sensory system to develop, he argues that it must have profound psycho-biological significance for normal behavioural and physical development. In addition to the evidence of abnormal development in animals deprived of touch, there is evidence of similar abnormalities in humans. Children raised by parents or others who for reasons of insensitivity, emotional instability, cruelty or belief, withhold contact (touching, stroking, fondling) and affection from them, exhibit abnormal psychological development. This may continue into adult life and be perpetuated on their own children. It is of interest that battering and abusing parents, treated similarly themselves as children, rarely report having a pet.

Montagu also refers to positive results of tactile contact in animals. For instance he comments that hand-milked cows give more and richer milk than machine-milked cows, that using touch to gentle young rats makes them better able to tolerate stressful situations as adults, and that dolphins like to be gently stroked.

CETACEA

In captivity, social interaction, including tactile contact between trainer and dolphin is standard practice and seen to be an important factor in bonding the relationship and developing good rapport. We know from trainers' and researchers' reports that such bonds can be unusually strong—more so than with other animals—and that separation can result in very stressful experiences for both trainer and dolphin (Lilly 1967).

There seems to be ample evidence now, and in any case it seems reasonable to extrapolate from the data on other highly evolved social animals (wolves, elephants, primates), that social interaction and tactile contact are of significant importance to many species of cetacea. We know, for example, that their skin is a highly refined sensory organ of touch and that in groups of whales and dolphins physical contact is necessary and frequent. As in the case of other animals, cetacea/human bonding seems to involve a mutual need for touching and stroking, and also seems to involve (at least, as observed in captivity) mutually strong emotional ties. It is well known that when captured or placed in stressful situations, dolphins respond well to human touch. Robson has commented that when touched and stroked and spoken to soothingly, stranded whales become calm and less stressed.

Animal/human bond research has in fact included work with captive dolphins. Henry Truby, one of John Lilly's colleagues, observed play interaction between neurologically impaired people and dolphins and concluded that they were mutually beneficial. More recently in

1978, Truby and Smith, a Florida researcher, started to explore whether captive dolphins could have a positive effect on the behaviour of autistic children. Infantile autism, characterized by delayed and deviant language development, severely impaired capacities to relate to people and objects, extreme withdrawal and failure to respond to sensory stimuli, is sometimes called a communication disease. Any modicum of success with these children can be regarded as a breakthrough.

In the Florida study with eight autistic children, all eight showed, amongst several behaviour improvements, unusually long attention spans. One boy, Michael, an 18 year old, fed fish to dolphins, poured water over them and made clicking noises to gain their attention. Not only was such interactive play behavior, that is reaching out beyond himself, highly unusual, but beyond speaking two words, he had never before made efforts at verbal communication. Smith reports not only temporary but sustained changes in his behaviour, namely, excitement on seeing dolphins, grabbing other people to indicate the dolphins, recognition of and clicking at dolphins on television and in books, and the use of the word "yep" five times in one week in response to questions about dolphin visits (Smith 1982).

There is as yet no available data on the dolphins' reaction to these children, but recognizing the intractable nature of this emotional disorder and the unusually positive results, interesting speculations might be made about the value of cetacea in this kind of work.

The literature indicates that cetaceans historically have demonstrated a benign interest towards us, and that, in the face of some of our worst atrocities. It further demonstrates a strong emotional pull towards cetaceans on the part of humans since the earliest times. Cetaceans have shown interest in us in a variety of ways. There are many examples of the lone dolphin establishing strong relationships with people in local waters, sometimes selecting particular individuals, often children, e.g., Opo and Horace in New Zealand, Donald in Britain, Jean Louis in France, and Sandy in the Bahamas. Wade Doak has collected hundreds of anecdotes from divers, sailors, long distance swimmers, surfers, etc., commenting on their dolphin encounters —playing, being protected from sharks, guided to safe waters, being accompanied, seeking contact, etc. (Doak 1981). Relatively recently scientists have become aware of a unique situation on the remote coast of Western Australia at Monkey Mia, where for the last 16 years a group of dolphins have been visiting the beach to interact with people. Fish are fed to the dolphins but there is also a great deal of tactile contact and vocal exchanges. While most scientists are convinced that the food reward is quite secondary to the importance of social interaction, no controlled studies have yet been carried out. The amount of reported evidence of even whales seeking contact with humans is increasing, e.g., humpbacks in Hawaii, greys in Mexico, sperm in New Zealand, and right whales in Patagonia.

There seems to be little doubt that tactile contact between humans and animals is not only mutually beneficial but also mutually pleasurable. Messent (1981) commented that in our society the need for tactile contact and the opportunity to satisfy it may have values we do not yet understand. It may well be that it is of paramount importance to us because it represents an outward expression of the emotion of love. Darwin (1955) in his book *The Expression of Emotions in Man and Animals* shocked the scientific community in 1872 with his claim that human expression of emotion, although more differentiated was similar if not identical to that in animals. Emotions were expressed in all creatures in a manner designed to effectively communicate to others what was being felt inside. He stated that the emotion of love was an exception to all the general rules in that while it was the most powerful of all emotions, it was the only one with no special means of expression:

> *Although the emotion of love, for instance that of a mother for her infant, is one of the strongest of which the mind is capable, it can hardly be said to have any proper or peculiar means of expression....A strong desire to touch the beloved person is commonly felt...love is expressed by this means more plainly than by any other....With the lower animals we see the same principle of pleasure derived from contact in association with love.*

DISCUSSION

While most of us would agree with Darwin that "the emotion of love...is one of the strongest of which the mind is capable," we also have to wonder why scientists in the twentieth century accepted Darwin's theories but almost totally neglected the study of the emotion he deemed most important.

The sensitivity of touch and its relationship to the emotion of love certainly raises some questions about both the importance of animals in our lives and the nature of animal emotion and consciousness. It also raises important questions about cetacea and our relationship with them. The history of close encounter with cetacea may not be accidental if Alistair Hardy is correct that we were once aquatic apes living in the shallows in close harmony and possibly close tactile contact with coastal cetacea, rather than in the prey/predator relationship as with most other animals (Morgan 1982).

Given the intelligence of dolphins, the innumerable instances of sensitive behaviour towards people and their affinity for children, the therapeutic benefit could be quite extraordinary. Particularly so since at the present time we do not know very much about the minds of other species and in what ways they communicate non-verbally, least of all about the big-brained acoustically oriented cetacea.

At least there now seems to be some shift away from our traditional arrogant and anthropocentric way of viewing animal behaviour. Scientists are considering heretofore heretical ideas about the intelligence, culture, language and consciousness of animals (Norris, Pribram, Terrace, J.J. Bonner, etc.). Speculation has it that some species of whales and dolphins might be able to transmit and interpret visual thought patterns. If there is any truth in this then therapeutic interaction with severely disturbed people, the blind, the deaf and others whose communication patterns are hindered, might be of primary importance.

While this author is not in favour of captivity, it nevertheless remains true that permits for capture are still being issued and that a number of cetaceans are now in captivity and will likely remain so for several more years. These social animals whose need for love and affection, social interaction and tactile contact may be no less than ours, and who have demonstrated over the centuries a desire to interact with humans, may benefit equally from therapeutic interactions. Such involvements may well outstrip any psychological benefits currently accruing from their involvement in cognitive research and entertainment.

While in some ways it seems less practical to involve wild cetaceans, it may become less so as: (a) the whale sighting tourist industry increases; and (b) reports of locations of friendly whales and dolphins increases. Again, and this is equally speculative, it may be that those amongst us, who for reasons of physical handicap or emotional trauma, chose or are forced to use uncommon modes of communication, could find meaningful affective communication with cetacea, as yet indecipherable to the rest of us in our logical linear world.

CONCLUSION

This evidence of mutual benefit from interaction is hardly surprising if we pause to think about our biological and evolutionary heritage, of the intricate interdependency between human and animal down the ages. It appears likely that the human/companion animal bond is of great antiquity beginning perhaps with man's capacity to reach out to the young of wild animals, culminating about 12,000 years ago in domestication of canids. It is clear that animals are still important to modern man—not just for material resources, when we consider that there are approximately 35 million dogs and 25 million cats in American households alone. In terms of our psychological development, the animal is a universal dream symbol, playing a powerful role, not only in our dreams, fantasies, folktales, art and religion, but in our neuroses and psychoses. Our children are said to first dream of animals (Levinson 1972).

However, an explanation of the evolution of our attitudes towards nature, in general, and animals in particular, reveals a relatively recent but ever increasing shift from cooperative interdependence to competitive independence, with an almost complete and arrogant disregard for our biopsychological kinship and needs. Much has been written on the demise of species and environments and possibly the planet itself under the domination of the human animal (e.g., Leiss 1974). While we have "successfully" domesticated nature, bringing it close to the brink of total disaster, it could clearly be argued that we have severely lost rather than gained in personal contentment, psychological stability and social cohesion—witness, for example, the human agony in our hospitals, mental institutions and prisons, and the perplexities and confusions in ourselves and our everyday lives.

Human-animal bond research with its rather ironic findings that not only do healthy people benefit from such a bond but that in some cases animal therapy is the only therapy to give any positive results, may help to provoke a much needed return to a respect for and a cooperation with other species, both wild and domestic.

Much has been written about species interdependency in terms of basic survival needs. Relatively little has been written about the possiblility of species interdependency at an emotional level. Involving cetaceans in therapeutic situations may usefully extend the range of human/animal bond research in ways which could be important to the mental and physical well being of many species, including humans. Considering the impressive results from therapeutic work with pets and domestic animals, how much more dramatic might the results of such work be with animals whose brain capacity is much close to our own?

We may even come to acknowledge a primary human need to live cooperatively with other species. Finally, in the ironic fact of their sometimes unique capacity to guide us back to sanity, we may also acknowledge their qualitatively equal differences and therefore their equal rights to survival.

REFERENCES

Adell-Bath, M., Krook, A., Sandquist, G., and Skantze, K. 1979. Do we need dogs? A study of dogs' social significance to man. University of Gothenburg.

Coelho, A.M. Jr. 1980. Guardian behavior by baboons towards felines. *Laboratory Primate Newsletter* 19:1-10.

Corson, S., O'Leary Corson, E., and Alexander, J.A. eds. 1980. *Ethology and nonverbal communication in mental health: An interdisciplinary biopsychosocial exploration.* London: Pergamon Press.

Darwin, C. 1955. *The expressions of the emotions in man and animals.* New York: Philosophical Library.

Doak, W. 1981. *Dolphin dolphin.* Auckland, N.Z.: Hodder & Stoughton.

Friedmann, E., Katcher, A.H., Lynch, J.J., and Thomas, S.A. 1980. Animal companions and one-year survival of patients after discharge from a coronary care unit. *Public Health Reports* 95(4, July-August):307-12.

Gantt, W.H., Newton, J.E.O., Royer, F.L. and Stephens, J.H., 1966. Effect of person. *Conditional Reflex* 1:18-34.

Katcher, A.H. 1981. Interaction between people and their pets—form and function. In Fogle, B. ed. *Interrelations between people and pets.* Springfield, Illinois: Chas. C. Thomas.

Katcher, A.H. and Friedmann, E. 1980. Potential health value of pet ownership. *The Compendium on Continuing Education* 11(2,February):117-21.

Leiss, W. 1972. *The domination of nature.* Boston: Beacon Press.

Levinson, B. 1971. Household pets in training schools serving delinquent children. *Psychological Reports* 28:475-81.

Levinson, B. 1972. *Pets and human development.* Springfield, Illinois: Chas. C. Thomas.

Levinson, B. 1978. Pets and personality development. *Psychological Reports* 42:1031-38.

Levinson, B. 1969. *Pet oriented child psychotherapy.* Springfield, Illinois: Chas. C. Thomas.

Lilly, J.C. 1967. *Mind of the dolphin.* New York: Avon Books.

Messent, P.R. 1982. Increase in people-people contacts through dogs as social catalysts. For presentation at 20th International Congress of Applied Psychology, Edinburgh, 28 July 1982, pp. 25-31.

Montagu, A. 1978. *Touching.* New York: Harper and Row.

Morgan, E. 1982. *The aquatic ape.* London, England: Souvenir Press Ltd.

Mugford, R.A. and M'Comisky, J. 1974. Some recent work on the psychotherapeutic value of cage birds with old people. In Anderson, R.S. ed. *Pet animals and society.* London: Bailliere Tindall.

Saul, L.J. 1962. Psychosocial medicine and observation of animals. *Psychosomatic medicine* 24(1):58-61.

Searles, H.F. 1960. *The nonhuman environment.* New York: International Universities Press, Inc.

Smith, B. 1982. Unpublished paper on animal therapy with autistic children. Paper presented to the Society for Comparative Animal Studies, Paris.

Suomi, S.J., Harlow, H.F. and McKinney, W.T., Jr. 1972. Monkey psychiatrists. *American Journal of Psychiatry* 128(8, February):41-46.

Part III
Animal Rights

LOGIC AND LIMITS OF ANIMAL LIBERATION

Edward R. Bennett

Department of Medical Microbiology
School of Veterinary Medicine
University of Georgia
Athens, GA 30605

INTRODUCTION

The current interest in treatment towards animals goes beyond the focus of isolated instances of brutality and encompasses the advocacy of significant changes in our traditional attitudes toward animals. In one year (1980) an estimated 2,054,281,000 hogs, beef, lamb, and poultry were raised on farms and slaughtered in the U.S.* (Agricultural Statistics 1981), and 1,653,385 laboratory animals were used by facilities registered with the United States Department of Agriculture (USDA 1974). Adding to this the number of related animal industries such as textiles, farm equipment manufacturing, cosmetics and drug industries, restaurants, and groceries, it is easy to appreciate the broad spectrum of changes which would result from significant changes in our relationship with animals. Since all individuals have an interaction with animals, at least by the animal products they choose to purchase (or not to purchase), there has been a proliferation of viewpoints concerning the treatment of animals. This paper will primarily consider Peter Singer's arguments presented in his book, *Animal Lib-*

*Number in thousands: hogs—97,174; cows and heifers—14,905; steers—16,059; bulls—679; sheep and lambs—5,742; total poultry—19,169,722.

eration (1975), because it is a popular thesis which is objective and logically derived.

DEFINITIONS

Before considering views about our treatment of animals, it will be helpful to define and document several key terms.

Speciesism

Speciesism is a term used by Singer (1975) to mean "...a prejudice or attitude of bias toward the interests of members of one's own species and against those of members of other species."

Pain

The common dictionary definition of pain is "a distressing sensation as of soreness or mental suffering as applied to humans and other animals." (*Oxford Universal Dictionary* 1955). When it is applied to lower invertebrates Singer (1975) says "most mollusks are such rudimentary beings that it is difficult to imagine them feeling pain, or having other mental states." As a logical philosopher Singer admits that it is not yet possible to determine a precise line between organisms that feel pain and those that do not, but as an advocate for animal liberation, Singer (1975) says that "...somewhere between a shrimp and an oyster seems as good a place to draw the line as any..."

Stress

Stress is often imprecisely used as a catch-all term for unknown factors which adversely affect an animal. A precise definition which has a physiologically measurable effect has been given by Hans Selye (1976). He defines stress as "the state manifested by a specific syndrome which consists of all the non-specifically induced changes within a biological system." The specific syndrome is called the General Adaptation Syndrome (G.A.S.) and consists of a specified alarm reaction, a stage of resistance, and a stage of exhaustion. The alarm reaction can be measured physiologically and consists of adrenocortical enlargement, atrophy of the thymicolymphatic organ and gastro-intestinal ulcers. So stress is the result of nonspecific factors that cause the G.A.S. This definition permits us to recognize stress and quantify it by measuring the alarm reaction. It is important to note that stress can be good or detrimental depending upon how the biological systems adapt to the detrimental effects of stress.

Equal Consideration

The concept of equal consideration is used by Singer to determine the parameters of acceptable treatment. "The basic principle of equality does not require equal or identical treatment, it does require equal consideration." (Singer 1975). Equal consideration is the result of recognizing that the fundamental common capacity between humans and animals is the capacity to suffer or feel pleasure. Singer (1975) quotes Jeremy Bentham, "The question is not can they (animals) reason? nor can they talk? but, can they suffer?" If equal consideration is given, then animals should not be subject to anymore suffering than we find permissible in humans. He goes on to state:

> *...if we consider it wrong to inflict that much pain on a baby for no good reason then we must, unless we are speciesists, consider it equally wrong to inflict the same amount of pain on a horse for no good reason* (Singer 1975, p. 16).

SINGER'S PHILOSOPHY OF ANIMAL LIBERATION

Singer (1975) states that animals and humans share the capacity to suffer pain or experience pleasure and that this capacity is the defining element that gives an individual interests: "The capacity for suffering and enjoyment is a prerequisite for having interests at all..." We can attempt to compare the amount of suffering or pleasure between species, but Singer (1975) admits that precise comparisons are difficult.

> *It is probably true that comparisons of suffering between members of different species cannot be made precisely, but precision is not essential* (p. 17).

Precision is not essential since a great amount of suffering will be eliminated even if a change in treatments is limited to comparisons of suffering which can be made with certainty. Our treatment of different species should not permit them to suffer any more than we allow for any one species. "No matter what the nature of the being, the principle of equality requires that its suffering be counted equally with like suffering" (Singer 1975). In Singer's theory the capacity to feel pain is the only factor which should be used to give equal consideration to individuals regardless of species. However, on the subject of killing, he allows other factors to influence the principle of equal consideration. He says that it is just as wrong to kill animals when under the same conditions, we would not kill humans. He makes the claim that:

> *Just as most humans are speciesists in their readiness to cause pain to animals when they would not cause a similar pain to humans for the same reason, so most humans are speciesists in their readiness to kill animals when they would not kill humans* (Singer 1975, p. 18).

But he does allow that factors such as "self-awareness, intelligence, the capacity for meaningful relations with others and so on...may be relevant to the question of taking life" (Singer 1975).

ARGUMENTS

Since there are many proponents of animal liberation, there are a number of arguments which lack logical theory, are based on misconceptions, and allude to anthropomorphism. Several examples can be cited in Jonny Frank's (1979) article on factory farming. Frank (1979) says that a baby pig "...suffers abuse just like its mother: within a day or two of birth, the young piglet has its ears knotched, its teeth clipped, its tail docked, and if male, is castrated as well." He never tries to compare the pain (if any) to pain in humans. Is ear knotching in the pig more painful than ear piercing in humans? When Frank (1979) states that pigs' teeth are clipped, he does not explain that only the sharp tips of these needle teeth are removed (Esminger 1970). He also fails to say that the reason the sharp teeth are clipped is to prevent injury to the other piglets and to the sow's udder (Esminger 1970). The fact that the piglets show no apparent signs of pain since they continue to nurse and fight with littermates (a normal pecking order behavior) makes it necessary for Frank (1979) to justify why he calls this practice abusive. A similar argument can be made for tail docking and castration.

Frank (1979) gives a romaticized view of a good non-abusive farm in his statement that "Only a few small dairy farms conform to the traditional pastoral scene, permitting the cows to graze in outdoor pastures during good weather." He makes no attempt to objectively evaluate the suffering an animal may have in confinement versus pasture. The fact that he envisions cattle grazing only in "good weather" reveals his affinity for emotion rather than detached reasoning.

Unbounded by logic Frank goes on to boldly delve into the inner psyche of a bovine and claims "...the separation of the calf from its mother causes psychological harm." This statement is "justified" in a footnote: "Mason visited calf barns and calves would attempt to 'suckle a finger, hand, or part of our clothing.' A farmer explained that they always do this because 'they want their mothers I guess.'" The farmer's statement hardly qualifies as expert analysis and does not justify the leap from the observation of suckling behavior to the assumption of psychological harm.

As an advocate of animal liberation, Singer (1975) also occasionally disregards his philosophical objectivity:

> *Flesh taints our meals. Disguise it as we may, the fact remains that the centerpiece of our dinner has come to us from the slaughterhouses, dripping blood. Untreated and unrefrigerated, it soon begins to putrefy and stink. When we eat it, it sits heavily in our stomachs, blocking our digestive process until, days later, we struggle to excrete it* (p. 183).

Singer (1975) does not justify how his perception of sauces or creative gourmet techniques constitutes a disguise for meat, not to mention the many times meat is served plain with decoratively styled vegetables. His reference to dripping blood may be symbolic. If not, he makes the common mistake of confusing blood with the inter- and extra-cellular fluid (not blood) that contains the pigment myoglobin, which reacts with oxygen and turns red. Any blood that still remained on the carcass would be coagulated by the time it leaves the slaughter house, and it would not be dripping. Since the decay to which Singer objects also occurs in fruits and vegetables, his comment is not a valid argument. Finally, to justify the statement that meat blocks our digestive system, Singer refers to research which compares the mean transit time of food moving through the digestive tract of nonvegetarians with that of vegetarians. Although there is speculation about the correlation between the increased transit time and increased incidence of colon cancer, the implication of this speculation, if it is correct, would not necessarily be that meat is bad but that the diet should contain more roughage.

There are a number of common objections that are made against Singer's theory of animal liberation, but the nature of the theory is such that most objections can be shown to deny equal consideration on the basis of irrational speciesism. The practical application of animal liberation would cause significant changes in the ways animals are raised on farms (if they are raised at all) and the use of animals in research. The objective of farm management like other businesses is to produce the maximum product (milk, eggs, meat, fiber) at the minimum cost. The criticism raised by animal liberationists is that equal consideration to the interests of animals is not a factor in farm management. The common objectives often raised by agricultural interests are: (Singer 1975)

1. Domestic animals are selectively bred by man for the purpose of farming so without agriculture the animals would not exist.
2. The farm animals were born and raised on a farm and have never known other conditions so they do not know what it means to live independently.
3. Conditions on the farm "...are no worse than conditions in the wild where animals are exposed to cold, hunger and predators."

Singer's reply to the first criticism is that "once a being exists, we have an obligation to avoid making that being suffer unnecessarily, but we have no obligation to nonexistent beings."

His response to the second criticism is that "animals feel a need to exercise, stretch their limbs or wings, groom themselves, and turn around, whether or not they have ever lived in conditions that permit this." (Singer 1975)

Singer (1975) answers the third criticism by saying that the choice "is not between life on a factory farm and life in the wild, but whether animals destined to live on factory farms and then be killed for food should be born at all."

Ewbank (1973) has attempted to classify groups of behavior changes that may be caused by intensive confinement management.

> Type I...abnormal behavior patterns are associated with pathological changes and obvious economic loss.
>
> Type II...abnormal behavioral patterns occurring with little or no evidence of economic loss.
>
> Type III...changes are qualitative alterations in otherwise normal behavioral patterns and are detectable only by systematic observation.

He says that it is difficult to assess the behavioral changes in Types II and III but says that Type I problems are "self-evident." Singer (1975) would believe that there could be significant changes in our treatment of animals even if we only considered the Type I behavior. He states:

> *Even if we were to prevent this infliction of suffering on animals only when it is quite certain that the interests of humans will not be affected to anything like the extent that animals are affected, we would be forced to make radical changes in our treatment of animals...* (p. 17).

ANIMAL RIGHTS

The debate about animal rights complicates the issue of animal liberation. We can classify two types of rights—legal and moral. We may define legal rights as those that society assigns while moral rights can be considered as those that society recognizes as inherent. According to Stone as reported by Dichter (1979) "...there is no generally accepted standard for legal rights..." But Stone (Dichter 1979) defines four conditions for having legal rights:

1. need an authoritative body to review and enforce rights,

2. must institute legal action at the animals' behest,
3. court must take injury into account,
4. relief must run to the benefit of the animal.

The definition of moral rights may cause more debate. One argument is that "animals are capable of suffering and of frustration and therefore have interests in the same manner that senile persons, infants, and brain damaged people have rights, even though they are intellectually deficient and cannot claim them." (*The Futurist* 1979) Singer (1975) also shares this view when he says "to avoid speciesism, we must allow that beings which are similar in all relevant respects have a similar right to life—and mere membership in our own biological species cannot be a morally relevant criterion for this right."

Michael A. Fox (1978) argues that since there are no "...attributes that all humans without exception share in common...even the capacity of humans to experience pain and pleasure falls short of universality...," we should "...shift our attention instead to capacities that are nearly or virtually universal among humans." By doing this we can find attributes that humans have and animals do not so Fox (1978) concludes "...that the concept of a moral right to equal treatment makes no sense except as applied to humans."

This argument misses the point of Singer's (1975) argument that the criterion is not a universal capacity for pain or pleasure within a species but that individuals, regardless of their species, that have the same capacity for pain or pleasure, should have equal consideration in treatment with respect to this capacity. Singer (1978) says:

> *I do not deny that normal human beings may possess capacities lacked by both retarded humans and animals. My point is that anyone wishing to defend our existing attitudes has to find some basis for attributing rights which does apply to all human beings but not to other animals. I claim that no such basis exists.*

To avoid this criticism, Fox (1978) adds an essential statement that "...autonomy, which thus entails certain cognitive capacities, is necessary (and, together with the capacity to enjoy or suffer, sufficient) for the possession of moral rights." Unfortunately, he does not give any justification for this point. "How can the above entailments be defended? I cannot give full treatment to this important argument here..." Without providing this justification Fox's theory is incomplete and fails to challenge Singer's argument.

OTHER ARGUMENTS

We may raise the question about our role in the naturally occurring predator-prey relationship which clearly violates the principle of equal consideration. Singer (1975) says we should not interfere because "...judging by our past record, any attempt to change ecological systems on a large scale is going to do far more harm than good." So apparently if there was a way to eliminate the actions of carnivorous species without causing major changes in the ecological balance, it would be justified.

A strong argument is to ask what animal liberationists plan to do about wild animals which feed on the plant crops. Singer's (1975) response is to suggest the hope that "we may eventually develop methods of limiting the numbers of those species whose interests are genuinely incompatible with our own." But the main point is that Singer's philosophy is utilitarian and permits killing animals, after giving equal consideration if there are conflicting interests. Nozick (1974) outlines these characteristics of utilitarian theory:

1. maximize happiness for all living beings,
2. stringent side constraints on what a human may do to another human and
3. animals may be used or sacrificed for the benefit of other people or animals only if those benefits are greater than the loss inflicted.

Singer assumes that those side constraints for human treatment are based on the capacity to suffer and should be applied among all individuals according to their capacity to suffer regardless of the species. But we may argue that those side constraints are based on other factors in addition to suffering.

As mentioned above Singer (1975) says that the factors such as "self-awareness, intelligence, the capacity for meaningful relations with others, and so on, are not relevant to the question of inflicting pain—since pain is pain,...these capacities may be relevant to the question of taking life." The reason that other capacities are permitted in the question of killing is because:

> *...people hold widely differing views about when it is legitimate to kill humans as the continuing debates over abortion and euthanasia attest. Nor have moral philosophers been able to agree on exactly what it is that makes it wrong to kill humans, and under what circumstances killing a human being may be justifiable* (Singer 1975, p. 18).

So the argument "pain is pain" cannot be countered by saying killing is killing since there are different factors which influence when killing may be morally justified in humans. The argument that the capacity to suffer is the only criterion to be used in equal consideration because "pain is pain," is justified by the assumption that people must hold a common view about when it is legitimate to cause pain in humans and that moral philosophers must be able to agree when pain is justified. Singer does not state this, but it is the logical parallel of his argument on killing applied to pain. This is the implied explanation for the statement "pain is pain." This is the fundamental point where we can raise strong objections to Singer's theory of animal liberation.

While Singer's theory is utilitarian with respect to killing animals, he assumes that there is a moral concensus on human suffering which is based only on the capacity to suffer and is free of other utilitarian factors. Singer would allow factors in addition to suffering in the debates about abortion or the death penalty since these topics involve the question of killing. But in subjects such as slavery or civil rights, Singer would hold that the only necessary factor is the amount of suffering. In this respect, Singer's theory is not utilitarian since it violates Nozick's (1974) third characteristic of a utilitarian position that "...animals may be used or sacrificed for the benefit of other people or animals only if those benefits are greater than the loss inflicted." It may be that Singer assumes that these other factors are used in determining treatment in humans, but he cannot simply give equal consideration to other species based only on the capacity to suffer because the amount of suffering was not the only factor considered in determining the moral standard of treatment in the first place.

Our treatment of other people is based on many factors, one of which is emotional attachment. We see this in animals with maternal attachment or rejection, and we observe it in humans by the intuitive observation that we are more sensitive to the pain or pleasure of people to whom we have closer psychological bonds. Just as we make emotional bonds to certain human individuals, we also make bonds to animals and this bond affects our treatment of them. "Although regarded as acceptable fare on the continent, eating horse meat is akin to cannibalism in Britain" (*The Economist* 1978). One reason that a laboratory animal which may have "a higher degree of self-awareness and a greater capacity for meaningful relations with others than a severely retarded infant" (Singer 1975), may still be used in research rather than the infant, is because there is a greater emotional attachment made to the infant. This theory is not speciesist since it also holds that it may be wrong to take someone's pet and use it in an experiment since there is an emotional bond made to the pet animal. Admittedly this factor elevates the human species since it always applies to humans and it is not always applicable to animals. However, it does not make the theory speciesist since it does not imply that only the presence or lack of emotional bond should determine treatment. It only suggests that other factors, in addition to the capacity to suffer, should influence our treatment of animals just as it influences treatment of other humans.

CONCLUSION

In the debate about animal liberation, it is necessary to define terms and focus on philosophically clear arguments which minimize casual inaccuracies and are free from emotional embellishment. We have considered Singer's theory of animal liberation and can conclude that to be acceptable, Singer must allow other factors in addition to suffering to directly influence equal consideration. It was argued that this can be done without resulting in speciesism. The practical application of the theory will still result in significant non-speciesist re-evaluation of treatment of animals.

REFERENCES

Agricultural Statistics 1981. United States Government Printing Office, Washington, D.C. 0-343-911.

Dichter, A. 1979. Legal definitions of cruelty and animal rights. *Boston College Environmental Affairs Law Review* 7:147-64.

The Economist. 1978. Eating pets is wrong. July 1:26.

Ensminger, M.E. 1970. *The Stockman's handbook.* Danville, Illinois:The Interstate Printers and Publishers, Inc.

Ewbank, R. 1973. The trouble with being a farm animal. *New Scientist* 18:172-3.

Fox, M.A. 1978. 'Animal liberation': A Critique. *Ethics* 88:106-18.

Frank, J. 1979. Factory farming: An imminent clash between animal rights activists and agribusiness. *Boston College Environmental Affairs Law Review* 7:423-61.

The Futurist. 1979. Rethinking animal rights. June:239.

Nozick, R. 1974. *Anarchy, state, and utopia.* New York:Basic Books, Inc.

Oxford Universal Dictionary, 1955. Third Edition.

Selye, H. 1976. *The stress of life.* New York:McGraw-Hill Book Co.

Singer, P. 1975. *Animal liberation.* New York:Avon Books.

__________. 1978. The fable of the fox and the unliberated animals. *Ethics* 88:120-1.

United States Department of Agriculture. June 1974. *Animal Welfare Enforcement.* 1973 Report of the Secretary of Agriculture to the President of the Senate and the Speaker of the House of Representatives:pp. 19-21.

WHALES ARE NOT CETACEAN RESOURCES*

Dale Jamieson† and Tom Regan‡

†*Department of Philosophy*
University of Colorado
Boulder, Colorado 80302

‡*Department of Philosophy and Religion*
North Carolina State University
Raleigh, North Carolina 27695

ABSTRACT

What we know about whales is sufficient for ascribing to them the analogues of human rights, including the fundamental right to be treated with respect. Once we recognize their possession of this right, it follows that whales are not to be used or exploited by us for the promotion of our ends, however "benign" they may appear. In the case of humans, to refrain from killing them is to discharge only a small part of our total duties. We must also refrain from exploiting them, whether "consumptively" or "nonconsumptively." Having come as far as we have in our understanding of the moral ties that binds humans and whales, we must now go further in our deeds. Just as whales are not here for us to kill for our purposes, so they are not here for us "to study," or "to watch," or "to play with." The moral task before us is the most difficult. It is to *let whales alone*.

---

*Presented to WHALES ALIVE: A Global Conference on the Nonconsumptive Utilization of Cetacean Resources, Boston, MA, 6 June 1983.

In 1946 representatives of fourteen governments met in Washington to sign the International Convention for the Regulation of Whaling. This was the meeting that established the International Whaling Commission. The declared purpose of the Convention was to safeguard the "great natural resources represented by whale stocks" in order to "make possible the orderly development of the whaling industry" (International Whaling Commission 1946).

Since 1946 attitudes towards whales have changed enormously both within the IWC and among the general world population. Public opinion surveys have indicated that in most countries, including Japan, opposition to whaling is the majority sentiment. The IWC, and especially its Scientific Committee, has reflected this shift in opinion, as well as playing a role in bringing it about. The Commission has contributed to our knowledge of whales by supporting the collection and collation of scientific data. This in turn has focused attention on the plight of the planet's largest mammals. In its 1980 Washington conference the IWC even began to explore tentatively the ethical issues involved in killing cetaceans. Today it seems to many that the IWC is as involved in protecting whales as in protecting the whaling industry. There seem to be at least two sources for this shift in attitudes towards whales.

First, recent research has suggested that whales are remarkably intelligent and sensitive creatures. Exactly how sensitive and intelligent, and how exactly these terms are to be applied to whales, is difficult to say, however. There are serious problems involved in studying whales. They live in very different environments than we do. The course of their evolutionary history has been very different, and there are also significant variations among species. Still, some things are known. Whales have extraordinarily large brains. Some have about 30 billion neurons in their neo-cortex compared to about 10 billion in humans. With brain to body ratios that are similar to those of the higher primates, their brains are also highly differentiated and exhibit a high degree of folding of the cortical surface. For these reasons one of the leading researchers in the field, P.J. Morgane, has claimed:

> *...only the brain of whales and men have the amount and quality of neocortex making both appear at the pinnacle of the animal kingdom...* (Frost 1979).

In addition, whales have extremely rich behavioral repertoires, sophisticated communication systems, and complex forms of social organization. Whatever finally may be decided about the exact nature of whale intelligence and sensitivity, it has become increasingly clear that whales are comparable to the higher primates and perhaps even to humans. For this reason it has seemed to many that killing whales for their blubber and oil is a moral crime akin or even equivalent to wanton murder.

A second reason why attitudes towards whales have changed is due to the apparent harmony in which whales live with their environment. Millions of years before our ancestors came out of the trees whales had already evolved to about their present state, and they were living lives very much like the ones they live today. For millions of years they were clearly the most intelligent beings on the planet. Seen from this perspective, we are evolutionary upstarts. In an incredibly short period of time we have become masters of the planet. And what do we do? We devote ourselves to destroying all other intelligent forms of life. But at least we are consistent. We seem just as willing to destroy ourselves as well. For people who despair at the havoc humans have wrought, whales are role models. They are symbols of how intelligent beings can live joyful, peaceful lives in harmony with their environment. From this point of view, whales are the teachers, we the students, about the things that really matter.

Whether or not we are willing to fully accept either of these lines of thought doesn't really matter. It is clear that we have all come a long way since 1946 in our attitudes towards whales. To some degree this Conference marks the progress we have made. Instead of talking about "maximum sustainable yields" we are now talking about "whales alive" and the "nonconsumptive utilization of cetacean resources."

In the light of the progress we have made it would be nice to say that we have gone far enough, that we are on the verge of a new era in which we give the whales their due. If this were the case, this Conference would be the occasion for a double celebration: one for the whales, and one for us for celebrating them. We shall argue, however, that although we have freed ourselves from the worst aspects of the anthropocentric ethic, which holds that everything on the planet only has value insofar as it has value to us—our ends, our purposes, our interests—we have not yet fully liberated ourselves from its lingering vestiges.

Not everyone will be willing to accept what we say. But whatever beliefs we finally come to, it is important that we be willing from time to time to reconsider them, and to scrutinize honestly the fundamental presuppositions and commitments on which they are based. We hope that this paper will be a contribution to such a reconsideration.

First we shall argue that what we know about whales is sufficient for ascribing to them the analogues of human rights, including a right to life, a right that is violated by those whaling practices that we are beginning to put behind us. We shall argue further that this right is undergirded by a more fundamental right that whales share with humans: a right to be treated with respect. It is this right which would be violated by allowing, for instance, exploitative benign research on humans. And it is this right that is violated when we treat whales as "cetacean resources." Next we shall discuss some of the implications of our view for the concerns of this Conference.

WHALE RIGHTS

To credit whales with a comparatively sophisticated mental life is hardly new. It is in the spirit of Darwin who claimed repeatedly that conciousness forms a continuum; the mental life of the higher animals differs from our own only in degree, not in kind. Any rationally viable ethic of how whales ought to be treated must take their mental sophistication into account. And it is the demonstrable failure to do this that exposes the grave inadequacy of the "ethic" that allows these animals to be viewed and treated as a resource for us, as if they were trees or mineral deposits. Just as Bonnie is not a resource for Clyde, nor Clyde for Bonnie, so whales are not a resource for us—though of course they can be, and almost always are, treated as if this is their "place in the scheme of things." That we are, so to speak, on all fours with whales on this morally crucial matter will be seen more clearly once we reflect on the philosophical underpinnings of why we do, and should, deny that human beings are to be viewed and treated as other peoples' resources.

In our case we avoid this impoverished view by postulating that we have a different kind of value. Sometimes this is said to be our worth, or our dignity, or our sanctity; sometimes, as in Kant's writings, the root idea is expressed by saying that human beings exist as "ends in themselves." That is to say, people as individuals have their own projects and purposes that imbue their lives with meaning. As a member of the human community I recognize that others have virtues and excellences which they strive to develop more fully. I may not share their conception of virtue and of the good, but I recognize that they, like me, have legitimate ends which they pursue, which are valuable to them, and so if I am to be moral I must treat them as independent beings with their own excellences—as "ends in themselves." Let us here call the kind of independent, nonresource value attributed to individual humans inherent value. It is because we have such value that we must not be treated in ways that fail to show respect for us as individuals, and respect is not shown whenever we are treated in ways that assume that our value is reducible to how much we answer to or advance the interests of others—as if, that is, we exist as a resource for others. Acts and institutions that fail to treat us with appropriate respect, from a deceitful promise to slavery, are to be morally condemned. Or so it is commonly believed. Were we to grant this much, how could we rationally avoid the same view about the value of whales, since they too seem to have their own virtues and excellences? How could we rationally defend, that is, the view that we have this special kind of nonresource value—inherent value—but they do not?

Many possibilities come to mind: Whales lack immortal souls. Whales lack moral autonomy and reason. Whales lack the ability to enter into contracts. Whales lack the ability to choose between alternative life-plans. And so on. Some of these claims are almost certainly false. But even if they are granted, for argument's sake, they neither singly nor collectively provide a rationally satisfactory basis for affirming inherent value in our case while denying it in the case of whales. For example, even if it is true that we do, but whales do not, have immortal souls, nothing whatever follows concerning the sort of value each of us has during our terrestial life. Again, that whales lack the ability to recognize the inherent value of others, should this be true, is no better reason to deny that they have such value than it would be to say that a daffodil cannot be yellow because it lacks the ability to recognize that lemons are yellow too. And as for the other sorts of considerations mentioned (for example, that whales lack, but humans possess, autonomy and reason), each conveniently overlooks the fact that *many* human beings who we regard as having inherent value—young children, the senile, and the mentally enfeebled, for example—are similarly deficient. We do not, and we should not, treat these human beings as if they exist as a resource for those of us who, as luck has it, happen to possess the list of favored attributes under review. To persist in viewing and treating whales, creatures who, it bears emphasizing, have a mental life of greater sophistication than many human beings, as if they exist as a resource *here for us*, their value to be measured in terms of how much they answer to and advance human interests, while denying that the same is true in the case of these humans—to persist in doing this is neither rationally nor morally defensible. Rationally, we are inconsistent in judging relevantly similar cases in dissimilar ways; morally, we are prejudiced because we draw moral boundaries on the basis of a biased consideration (namely, species membership), a tragic moral failing in the case of our dealings with animals that is not unlike other failings, such as racism and sexism, in our dealings with one another. For just as the moral status and value of a human being does not turn on such biological considerations as race or sex, so the moral status and value of an individual, whether human or cetacean, does not turn on the different biological consideration of species membership.

There is an obvious way around these charges of prejudice and inconsistency: give up the belief in our own inherent value. This is an option that will tempt some, but few on reflection will give in. And that is a good thing too. For the moral theory we would be obliged to put in the place of one that recognizes *our* independent, nonresource value will prove to be weak at the joints, unable to stand up under the weight of sustained, fair, and informed criticism (Regan 1983). So we do well not to make a shambles of our theoretical understanding of *interhuman* right and wrong in order to avoid recognizing our prejudice and inconsistency when it comes to the value of individuals beyond our species' borders. We do well, that is, to expand our moral vision rather than to close our eyes to our human fallibilities.

The inherent, nonresource value of a human being is the linchpin of the idea that individual human beings have *basic moral rights*, including such rights as the rights to life, to liberty, and to privacy. If Jack is to show respect for Jill's inherent value, he is obliged to respect her rights; he must not do anything to her that reduces her status in the world to that of a mere resource for others. Thus must he not kill her, for example, so that he, or his children, or the chronically destitute can have more of what they want or need; nor may he limit her freedom or invade her privacy just because he or others stand to reap some benefits, whether the benefits be monetary, recreational, or scientific. To recognize the inherent value and basic moral rights of a human being is to accept the *moral* inviolability of the individual. Like "No Trespass" signs, our basic rights mark off the boundaries of that unique "moral space" which, as individuals, we each occupy.

These same signs come into view once we accept the inherent, nonresource value of whales—and, with this, their basic rights. This is not to say that they do or must have *every* right a human being has—the right to vote, for example, or the right to attend the church of their choice. The basic rights they *do* have are those they *can* have. These include the ones mentioned earlier—rights to liberty, to privacy, to life, and to pursue their own wellbeing or happiness, all violated in a flash, one might say, when whales are killed for their meat or blubber, their oil or bone. But are any of these rights violated when, as many aspire to, we view and treat whales as objects that satisfy and advance our scientific, recreational, or, in either case, our economic interests? That is the central question that remains to be considered.

WHALE WRONGS

Let us consider the recreational uses of whales first. One way that people use whales for recreational purposes is by observing them in their natural habitat. Each winter in California, for example, thousands of people view the gray whale migration. Whales and other cetaceans are also kept in captivity so that they can be used for recreational purposes. Aquatic parks like Seaworld and Marineland train cetaceans to perform tricks for the pleasure of paying customers.

In the previous section we said that if whales have rights then they must be treated with respect. Their value and dignity does not rest on their place in our plans, purposes and projects. From this perspective our exploitation of whales for recreational purposes is not morally acceptable. They are not nature's toys to be "oohed" and "aahed" at by humans. They are not human artifacts made by us to fulfill our intentions. They are creatures of inherent value with lives of their own and the capacity to lead them in their own ways. To confine them in aquatic parks and to make them perform tricks that people find amusing is to try to remake them into our own creations. This attempt to appropriate such marvelous and magnificent creatures for such trivial purposes, denying them their liberty in the bargain, is morally to be condemned.

The commercial whale-watching industry—often viewed as the "benign" substitute for commercial whaling—is similarly unacceptable, though for a different reason. Whales do not exist as visual commodities in an aquatic free market, and the business of taking eager paying sightseers into their waters, though nonconsumptive, is exploitative nonetheless, morally analogous to making a business of conducting sightseeing tours of human beings who either cannot or do not give their consent to be exploited by other people in this way. Moreover, just as Grayline Tours of the black ghetto, or the barrio, or the gay community would tend to dehumanize and trivialize those whose very lives were being regarded as objects of curiosity and amusement, so it is also true in the case of the whales.

The "nonconsumptive uses" of whales for scientific purposes are extremely diverse. They include observing them in aerial surveys, recording their sounds, taking samples of tissues and fluids, and observing their behavior while held in captivity. Though "nonconsumptive," all too often whales are again directly treated as means to our ends. They are studied to satisfy *our* scientific curiosity or to test *our* scientific theories. Even so apparently harmless an activity as aerial viewing for purposes of population estimates should not completely escape moral skepticism, if the object is to determine whether a given species is at risk of extinction. Such studies foster, and are often in the service of, a false understanding of whales—as if, for example, the death of a whale matters only when a species is endangered. As with humans, so also with whales, it is individuals, not species, who have rights. We must take care not to accept that science that smothers the individual whale in numbers, graphs, charts, and so on. And we must also free ourselves from those enterprises that help perpetuate the general view that whales exist as one or another kind of resource, to be thought of in terms of "herds" or "stocks." To the extent that population and migratory studies are cut from this cloth, to that extent, and for that reason, they are wrong (Jamieson and Regan 1982; Regan 1983).

In defense of research on captive cetaceans it will be said that we overlook the many benefits, both real and potential, that have and will accrue for the animals themselves as a result of our scientific understanding of them. We have learned something about the maladies of cetaceans in captivity and as a result of this we are now better able both to prevent and cure them in the case of those animals now in our care. Like all benefits, however, the morality of those in question depends on the means used to secure them. And no benefits are morally to be allowed if they are obtained at the price of violating individual rights. Because, then, keeping these animals in captivity violates their rights, the gains obtained for whales and other cetaceans are ill-gotten. To take the rights of an individual whale seriously is to believe that individual whales no more exist as a source of benefits for other whales than they do for us.

Two kinds of response might be given to our argument. First, it is often said by people who work with whales and dolphins that these animals enjoy their interactions with humans, even those in experimental settings. Just as people like observing whales, so whales enjoy observing people. If this is correct then perhaps it can be said that in many cases whales "consent," in some sense, to be the subjects of benign research and to be entertainers in aquatic parks. If this is true then such "nonconsumptive uses" do not harm them, or if they do harm them, they do not violate their rights. It is difficult to know what to make of this claim. We should remember, however, that similar claims have often been made about oppressed humans as well as about other animals. It was said in defense of slavery that blacks enjoyed picking cotton and being taken care of by the master. It was said in defense of sexism that women preferred to stay home and do housework, and not compete in the cutthroat male world. Frequently today we see television commercials depicting happy cows and chickens, more than eager to lay down their lives for the sake of our palates. Perhaps these claims about the voluntary cooperation of cetaceans are true, but in the light of this history we should be highly skeptical. It is extremely doubtful that we add anything to the quality of cetacean life by our presence, more than doubtful that our absence would be missed by them.

The second response is that the "nonconsumptive use" of whales is important, because the whales themselves are the main beneficiaries of increases in our knowledge. This argument takes two forms.

The first claims that as a matter of *realpolitik*, whales will be killed as long as it is economically profitable to do so. If it can be shown that "nonconsumptive uses" of whales are economically preferable, then whaling will cease. There are a number of problems with this argument. First, it presupposes that "consumptive" and "nonconsumptive" uses of whales are mutually exclusive. James E. Scarff has argued that this is not the case (Scarff 1980). He cites as an example the fact that the Russians kill various numbers of gray whales every year in the Artic Ocean, without any apparent effect on the California whale-watching industry, even though both industries exploit the same species of whale. This suggests that nonconsumptive uses could simply add to rather than subtract from our repertoire of cetacean exploitation. But second, *realpolitik* is, so to speak, a two-edged sword. Even if it can be shown that whaling is an economically inferior use of whales relative to "nonconsumptive" uses, that still would not put the anti-whaling position on a firm foundation, since to accept the argument in this form suggests that whaling *should* continue if it can be shown to be the economically optimal use of whales. And while whaling may not be economically optimal now that whale populations are so low, there is no guarantee that the economic equation won't change in the future. The basic problem with this argument is, then, that it is analogous to saying that the reason we ought not to kill derelicts is because it is not economically efficient to do so. One would have thought the reason against this has *nothing whatever* to do with dollars and cents; and this is what we have argued is true of whales as well.

The second form of this argument suggests that the more we learn about whales the better able we will be to protect them. This argument undoubtedly has merit. We would not be in a position today to argue for the rights of whales were it not for the scientific research that has been done. And if we could be certain that additional benign research would redound to the benefit of the whales, who could oppose it? But again, history provides reason for skepticism. Sad though it is to say, science has been more often used against animals than for them. In the past we mainly have studied animals in order to make them a better resource rather than to ensure that they have better lives. By its very nature scientific knowledge is public information, and scientists are not in a position to control its uses. Sidney Holt has given one such example in which the results of benign research involving wolves is now being used against them (Global Conference on Non-Consumptive Utilization of Cetacean Resources 1983). Who can have confidence that this will not be the case with the whales as well? Even if we are motivated to do benign research on whales by the desire to improve their lot, we should be skeptical of our ability to do that. We have learned over and over again that human intervention in complicated natural systems often only makes things worse. Trying to be friends of the whales may only be another way of making us their enemies.

What we owe the whales is the recognition that they too are the bearers of moral rights, worthy of our respect. Once we are willing to accept, as we should, the idea that whales have the right not to be killed or needlessly harmed, consistency demands that we then acknowledge that they also have the right not to be exploited for the promotion of our ends, however "benign" they might appear, whether such exploitation is "consumptive" or "nonconsumptive." Having come as far as we have in understanding the moral ties that bind humans and whales, we must now go further in our deeds. Just as whales are not here for us to kill for our purposes, so they are not here for us "to study," or "to watch," or "to play with." The moral task before us is the most difficult because the most hidden and possibly self-sacrificial: It is to *let whales alone*, satisfied with the mere knowledge that these "other nations" continue to roam the vast reaches of the oceans in no small measure because of our principled efforts to save and preserve them.

REFERENCES

Frost, Sir Sidney 1979. *The Whaling Question* (The Inquiry by Sidney Frost of Australia), San Francisco: Friends of the Earth, p. 152.

Global Conference on Non-Consumptive Utilization of Cetacean Resources. 1983. 'Whales are not cetacean resources': Introductory Note. Boston, MA.

International Whaling Commission. 1946. *The International Convention for the Regulation of Whaling.* IWC, The Red House, Station Road., Histon, Cambridge, England, CB4 4NP.

Jamieson, D., and Regan, T. 1982. On the ethics of the use of animals in science. In: Regan, T. and VanDeVeer, D. eds. *And justice for all: New introductory essays in ethics and public policy.* Totowa, New Jersey: Rowman and Littlefield.

Regan, T. 1983. *The case for animal rights.* University of California: Berkeley Press.

Scarff, J.C. 1980. Ethical issues in whale and small cetacean management. *Environmental Ethics* 2(Fall):241–79.

Part IV
Animal Management

ANIMAL BOREDOM: IS A SCIENTIFIC STUDY OF THE SUBJECTIVE EXPERIENCES OF ANIMALS POSSIBLE?

Francoise Wemelsfelder

Instituut voor Theoretische Biologie
Groenhovenstraat 5, 2311 BT Leiden
Holland

INTRODUCTION

The study of animal well-being has now become an accepted field of scientific research. Until recently the dominant belief was that subjective experience was inaccessible to the natural sciences, since it could not be experimentally manipulated. It led so-called behaviourists to the denial of any sort of subjective life to animals. This scientific conception of animals is far removed from daily reality, in which people regard and treat animals as sentient beings. Second, the way we as human beings exploit animals for our own sake and profit has caused protest from several groups of people who consider these practices irresponsible and uncaring. Pigs, calves and chickens are "produced" in great quantity in small housing systems for meat consumption; rats and other species are extensively used in experimental laboratories, and all kinds of wild species are kept and bred in zoos. The will to improve the conditions in which these animals live has led to the development of a new field of scientific research: the science of animal welfare.

Marian Dawkins' book *Animal Suffering* (1980) gives an overview of current theories and problems, and it becomes apparent how difficult it is to find parameters for well-being which are truly adequate, insofar that we can be sure that certain parameters are directly representative of the limits within which animal well-being can exist.

Another, closely related field which has recently started to attract attention is the study of animal awareness or intelligence. D.R. Griffin's *The Question of Animal Awareness* (1981a) is the first book dealing extensively with the subject. Here too, it becomes clear how hard it is to relate criteria such as communicative ability, or adaptive behaviour to the existence of real understanding and awareness within the animal. What is the final discriminative evidence to distinguish "hard-wired" behaviour from intelligent behaviour, or an "instinctive" reaction from a really "felt" reaction? The question whether it is possible to study animal well-being scientifically therefore largely comes down to the question how we can bridge the "communication gap" between man and animal, or how we can become sure that what are usually considered to be indirect parameters are in fact direct.

This question has intrigued me for several years. In discussions with colleagues about the justifiability of vivisection, the argument whether or not animals can feel and suffer played a large role. The fact that something which seemed so obviously true to me was not accepted within a scientific framework and might even be inassessable that way puzzled me. I started to study literature on the phenomenon of pain in animals, since pain is biologically functional, and often overtly expressed; yet it also implies a purely subjective experience within the animal. It seemed to me that pain is a form of subjective feeling which (nevertheless) might be accessible to biological research. I explored this in an ethological research project on pain in piglets after castration without anaesthesia (Wemelsfelder 1982). It appeared that behavioural criteria rather than physiological ones are adequate to study pain, since behaviour represents the self-expression of the animal as an intrinsic whole, including any subjective experience it has. Physiological criteria seem to be more *in*directly linked to subjective experience.

However, current scientific methodology regards the reduction of phenomena to lower hierarchical levels as fundamentally desirable, and further there is the great danger of anthropomorphic interpretation of behaviour. Because of these reasons many scientists prefer physiological criteria on principle.

In fact, the importance which is attributed to different parameters or criteria seems to depend on the concept of scientific objectivity *itself*. Science is not the experience of reality as such; it constructs a *representation* of reality, and therefore the decision which representations of reality are valid and which are not so valid depends on the choice of a *meta*-scientific framework.

The aim of this paper is to explore the relationship between different meta-scientific frameworks and the science of animal welfare.

During the past few years, I have become more and more convinced that the great difficulty science has in studying subjective experience in its objects, might be related to the denial of any role to subjective experience in the *observer* as an interpretational guide. Can a quality in the world around us be observed, when this same quality is deliberately *ex*cluded from the process of observing?

As a practical example for the discussion described above, the phenomenon of animal boredom has been chosen. Boredom implies some sort of awareness, some form of a direct inner experience of selfhood. Because without a sense of selfhood related to the developmental potential of the animal, it would be impossible to "miss" certain things, to be bored. With the phenomenon of boredom one can illustrate the qualitative difference between behavioural and physiological deviations, but is still bored, since it misses the opportunity to perform its specific behaviour. How important behaviour is for an animal is a crucial question in theories on adaptation and stress, and as we shall see, on the existence of animal boredom as well.

Besides the fact that boredom is, theoretically speaking, an appropriate topic for a discussion about the possibility of studying animal welfare scientifically, it is also said to be a major problem for animals in intensive production systems (or bio-industry) and zoos, and in many cases in laboratories as well (van Putten 1982b; Markowitz 1982; Fox 1974). However, many people, farmers and scientists alike, share the view that when animals "are well fed, well watered and the temperature is very comfortable, I do not know what else you could do" (Kirkeide, Secretary of the North Dakota Beef Cattle Improvement Association, in the *Grand Forks Herald*, Nov. 28, 1982). It seems to be in the interest of the animals, therefore, to discuss whether boredom is a real problem which should be taken seriously, and how we might study and alleviate it if it is a problem and not some erroneous anthropomorphic inference.

Within the framework of the discussion mentioned above the following questions are central in this paper:

1. Can animals be bored, and what are important criteria in the study of boredom?
2. Is there evidence of boredom in intensive animal husbandry?

"OBJECTIVE" SCIENCE AND THE STUDY OF ANIMAL WELFARE

It has often been said that the study of the subjective is unscientific: inner, personal experiences are private and not accessible to methodological observation. In the science of psychology, verbal communication between observer and observed bridges most of the gap. In studying animals, however, this way of having access to their inner experience is closed. This dualistic view can be traced back to Descartes' well-known statement that "not only do animals have less reason than humans, they have none at all" (Gilson 1976). The idea that animals *are* mere material automata, not possessing any of the human "non-material" qualities, has since become quite influential. Yet it is *not a logical and necessary* conclusion.

To conclude that animals have no inner experience since it is not observable using the scientific method is only justifiable *within* the framework of the method used for observation. But it is not right to exclude the possibility *a priori* that the subjective world of animals could be observed and studied with other methods. What is presently accepted as "the scientific method" is not the only absolute guarantee for "objectivity," meaning complete knowledge of an object. Scientific ideas must ultimately be compatible with "common sense," or the common experience of humanity as a whole; with "those presumptions, which, in spite of criticism, we still employ for the regulation of our lives" (Whitehead, cited by Griffin 1977). The natural sciences, excluding inner experience (of animals, and humans as well since behaviorism) from their range of vision, are *not* compatible with human "common experience." Therefore it might be justifiable to say that current science represents *a choice* for a certain kind of relationship with the world; a relationship characterized by duality and total detachment between observer and observed, subject and object.

As a consequence of this duality, life has been reduced to material mechanisms; the natural sciences have become reductionistic in principle, with the science of Newtonian (mechanistic) physics at the basis of other, "derived" fields of study (Verhoog 1983).

It is possible, however, to think of a concept of "science" in which the *methodological* criteria for objectivity are maintained, but in which the *ontological* starting point is different from the current one. Tranoy (1977) makes this distinction between the two sorts of objectivity, and argues that ontological objectivity, implying a separation between object and subject, is "not universally acceptable..., not even reasonably uncontroversial." Furthermore, it has the serious limitation of excluding objects that are related to "subject-consciousness," like intentions, norms, feelings, etc. On the other hand, he says methodological objectivity is far more essential for any concept of knowledge. This implies conditions like intersubjectivity and consensus, sincere interest in an object, the absence of arbitrariness, etc. And, as has been said above, a concept of science which is consistent in this methodological sense, but is based on a non-dualistic ontological starting point (with emphasis on interconnectedness and interdependence) is very well possible.

The field of animal welfare is pre-eminently one in which different interests are likely to underly the different opinions on the matter. Between economic interests and the interests of the animal, scientific research is supposed to take a neutral position. The role of different scientific concepts in present controversies will now be examined.

Within the study of animal welfare, the subjective experience of the animals of course plays a crucial role. Welfare is in essence a subjective concept, and in order to study welfare, we should study the subjective world of an animal. Almost all natural scientists, however, agree that it is not possible to do experiments to demonstrate (prove) the existence of animal awareness and feeling. Analogy with humans or introspection are considered to be necessary to bridge the gap between outward behaviour and inner feeling, and many researchers are reluctant to do so through fear of anthropomorphism. One even says that "this idle speculation is a burdensome appendage to the real scientific work of observing and accounting for lawfulness in animal behaviour" (Zuriff 1982).

It may well be possible, however, to get access to this very important part of reality. "It is especially in the relationship human-animal (in which the duality object-subject is transcended) that animal consciousness can be best understood...and investigated" (Fox 1983b). Suffering is in principle such an intensely personal phenomenon (Cassel 1982) that it certainly cannot be studied in terms of "lawfulness." It requires willingness of individual observers to interpret data in an empathetic way. After a symposium on animal awareness Wood-Gush (1981) commented: "The general opinion seems to be that it (animal awareness) is very difficult to prove or disprove. The decision one takes is very much dependent on one's sympathy or attitude towards animals."

Those who have an economic interest in animals, accepting their exploitation for our benefit, have a different perspective on and interpretation of the situation than public groups, for instance, whose interest it is to assure the total well-being of the animal. The first group might state: "To exclude animals from fulfilling their role in helping to sustain the human population...is untenable" (American Society of Agricultural Engineers 1981). This point of view is accompanied by the notion that the general public should be informed "of the generally high level of animal care and husbandry exercised on most farms today, whether 'large or small'," since "their perceptions of animals are often unrealistic (oriented to Disney characters, pastoral scenes, and pets)" (ASAE 1981). Furthermore, it is believed that one of the negative aspects of "the current controversy on animal welfare" is that it is retarding the movement towards modern "technology which improves production."

Starting from the basic belief that animals exist to serve mankind, the main focus is upon production and efficiency, which at the same time seems to imply a belief that animal welfare in current systems is only marginally, not fundamentally, affected, and that people who think otherwise are sentimental and childish.

People whose primary interest is not to make money for a living by means of animal exploitation, have a totally different opinion; not because they are childish or sentimental, nor are their opinions "unscientific." They speak from the notion of "potential action." Regardless of any facts, we can give animals better housing than they have now, and make them less "unhappy." Ethical responsibility is more fundamental than scientific knowledge, as has been argued before, and therefore to consider nonscientists as "dumb crowds" is a misinterpretation of the fact that "man is a doer, not a knower" (Cave 1982; Debrock 1982). Scientific research in the sense of systematic observation can study different possibilities for reaching a desired goal, and so be a very important tool in making sure that our human ideas are reasonable, and correspond to natural reality.

Many animal-welfare scientists, however, think of the relationship between science and ethics in the opposite way: "The decisions whether or not we exploit animals...and to what extent,...are ethical decisions...that should be made by society at large,...but not without knowing the facts, or scientific evidence, provided by scientific research" (Duncan 1981). This statement can be said to represent the currently accepted view, in which ethical decisions are based on "objective" data. This statement obscures the fact that it is not always easy to discover hard scientific "fact." An interesting example is the phenomenon of adaptation, on which much research is focussed. An animal has to adapt to adverse situations, otherwise it dies. It does so by abnormal behaviour, for example. The question is, does an adapted animal suffer, or does "adapted" imply a calmed-down, relatively content animal? The first answer can be defended from a point of view in which the animal and its environment are seen as a meaningful whole, combined with empathetic observation of behaviour; the second can be defended by saying that behaviour is a stimulus-response mechanism, in which energy outlet is more important than the adequacy of the stimulus. So it seems that there is no "fact" here; the conclusion depends on which point of view one takes. This example will be discussed more elaborately in part I of this paper.

A "vice" that scientists often warn of or complain about is the danger of "anthropomorphic" thinking and reasoning, especially by non-scientifically trained people. But respect, involvement, care, and responsibility as integral parts of compassionate stewardship do not necessarily imply sentimental projection. The care is for the animal, and to fulfill *its* needs, rather than ours. To say that "a pig does not bathe in the mud because it likes it, but because it increases its possibilities for cutaneous evaporation" (Dantzler and Mormède 1979), is a denial of the subjectivity of the animal, and creates the duality between subjectivity and objectivity typical of scientific reductionism. The fear of anthropomorphism might well be a result of fear of taking animals completely seriously as fellow living beings; and for the "burden" of responsibility that would exist if it was accepted that our anthropomorphic notions about animals might be correct.

Biological data relevant to the concept of animal boredom will now be presented and discussed. In doing so, the ontological starting point of nondualism and empathic connectedness as developed in this introduction will be used as a basis. An attitude of empathy, serving as interpretational guideline, might give rise to controversial conclusions in the eyes of those who believe in a dualistic perspective. If it has been argued correctly that the choice of an attitude is primordial to observation, philosophically speaking, and that this choice directs the search for "scientific evidence," then the proposed procedure is justified.

PART I

ENVIRONMENTAL DEPRIVATION AND THE CONSEQUENCES FOR THE ANIMAL

The environment provides adequate stimuli to fulfill an animal's needs, and elicits appropriate, species-specific behaviour in an animal. In a diverse, rich environment, an animal has to search for these adequate stimuli (van Putten 1981). In a monotonous, "barren" environment, the animal is not only prohibited from searching for adequate stimuli most of the time, but hardly any adequate stimuli are present. This change in environment has an effect on the behaviour of the animal. What are these effects, and do they matter to an animal? In other words, does a change in quality of the environment affect the quality of the animal's life in a noticeable way for the animal?

DOES BEHAVIOUR MATTTER TO AN ANIMAL?

Behaviour includes all those processes by which an animal senses the external world and the internal state of its body, and responds to changes which it perceives (Manning 1972). Van den Assem (1973) adds that the term behaviour refers only to outwardly observable, mainly motor responses. In the course of time, several explanatory models for behaviour have been presented, which try to reduce behaviour "to a system of hypothetical components" (Manning 1972); components that are linked together in such a way that behaviour can be consistently predicted from certain conditions. "...ultimately we shall hope to explain behaviour in terms of the functioning of the basic units of the nervous system" (Manning 1972).

The question is, in this framework, where and how subjective experience fits into these kinds of models, and in what way an animal experiences its own behaviour.

In relation to the welfare of individual animals in a deprived environment, Hughes (1980) proposes a behavioural model which is an integration of the Lorenzian psychohydraulic model and the mixed-motivation model as developed by Deutsch and Hinde. The first states that behaviour is mainly caused by internal, genetic drives which have to be expressed, even if no adequate stimuli are present; the second model implies that behaviour is mainly triggered by external stimuli in combination with internal, chemical receptors, and, therefore, not performing a certain behaviour does not frustrate the animal. Hughes combines these two into a continuum: some behaviour patterns are mostly internally originated, some largely externally, and many arise through the interaction of rhythmically varying internal motivations and external releasers. In this framework the appearance of distorted or abnormal behaviour in a barren environment is clear evidence of a need for some environmental improvement, so he suggests, since the internal drive apparently is so strong that the absence of adequate releasing stimuli does not prevent an animal from performing abnormal behaviour.

This split into internally and externally regulated behaviour implies that not performing externally regulated behaviour in case of absence of stimuli may not be adverse to an animal. Or, an animal does not miss what it does not know, in other words.

How does an animal experience internally regulated behaviour that becomes distorted for lack of adequate stimuli? Any lack of an adequate environment requires adaptation of the animal to the present conditions. Adaptation is a fundamental property of each animal (Freeman 1975), and "basically all behaviours, including disturbed ones, represent adaptations of an organism to its '*Umwelt*'" (Wiepkema 1982).

Proposing a model for adaptive behaviour, Wiepkema (1980) uses the terms "*soll-werte*" and "*ist-werte*," meaning, respectively, the way an animal expects its environment to be and the way its environment actually is perceived to be. When there is a difference between *soll-werte* and *ist-werte*, the animal makes, or tries to make the required behavioural or physiological adjustments in order to solve the conflict. If the gap is too big, however, "abnormal" behaviour is a sign of the difficulty the animal experiences in attempting to control its environment adequately. According to Wiepkema, abnormal adjustments are accompanied by emotions such as fear and general suffering. After a certain time, when the animal has not been able to regain satisfactory control, the physiological parameters revert to apparent normality, and conflict behaviour develops into stereotypic behaviours. These stereotypic behaviours are not necessarily adverse anymore; on the contrary, they might *prevent* the animal from feeling unhappy, by calming the animal down and suggesting restored controllability (Wiepkema 1982). Discussing Lorenz's psychohydraulic model, Duncan (1981) says that "even if a psychohydraulic model is accepted, it could be argued that as long as the energy finds an outlet (into abnormal behaviour—*au*) that is not damaging to the hen itself or its flockmates, then welfare will not be adversely affected."

From the models presented above, we could conclude that not performing (potential) behaviour does not matter to an animal; that abnormal behavioural adjustments do matter to animals initially; but that more permanent abnormal behaviour might not be adverse anymore.

This way of looking at an animal and its behaviour, however, is the result of a reductionistic approach: the starting point is a dualistic perspective of animal versus environment, internal versus external. Wanting to reduce behaviour to neural systems (Manning 1972) may imply the view that the subjective experience of an animal is only secondarily, temporarily present.

In a recent article, Baxter (1982/83) gives an analysis of functional behaviour in relation to animal production and welfare, which could illustrate this way of thinking somewhat further.

He states that only those species-specific behaviour patterns which promote biological fitness have survived the pressure of natural selection. By biological fitness is meant reproductive potential, and all factors that contribute to this, such as number and quality of offspring, ability to rear offspring, etc. Subjective well-being therefore must also have some function towards this goal, and "will have been selected on the basis of its *representation* of biological fitness." Brain programs cause "the animal to change its current state by inducing pleasurable or displeasurable sensations...The study of animal welfare becomes therefore the study of the programs of their brains."

From this perspective he proceeds to say that the *consequences* of behaviour are crucial for animal productivity, and therefore for their welfare, rather than the behaviour itself: "allowing an animal to perform behaviour is one way of accommodating requirements, and is not the requirement itself....This opens the possibility of accommodating animal requirements entirely by environmental manipulation and without the animal performing behaviour." Ethology in this framework becomes an attempt at functional interpretation of behaviour, rather than a study of behavioural requirements in their own rights.

In short, subjective experience, and behaviour are said to be *secondary means* towards the goal of (re)production. The motor which moves the different parts of the mechanism is the central nervous system. And, as Ingram (1981) comments: "if an animal survives so that its DNA gets into the next generation, it has been a success."

These perspectives on behaviour do not regard animals as individual, qualitative, sensitive beings, but as mechanisms which find their reason for existence in quantitative production.

From a nondualistic perspective in which qualitative relationships are crucial for the animal's well-being it *does* matter to an animal when it does not have the chance to perform the behaviour which is part of a species-specific range of behavioural possibilities. The behavioural potential of an animal represents the quality of the animal-environment relationship. Rather than regarding behaviour as a means towards reproduction (in other words quality serving quantity), a nondualistic perspective regards reproduction as *a means towards individual life and behaviour* (quantity serving quality). Subjective experience is intrinsically present in all activity and together with behavioural expression represents the meaningfulness, the telos, of animal life.

In this way, distorted abnormal behaviour is an indication of an affliction upon the quality of the animal's life. What follows is a further discussion of abnormal behaviour, its forms of appearance and function.

The types of abnormal behaviour which occur mostly in barren, deprived environments are stereotypic behaviour, redirected behaviour, vacuum behaviour (van Putten 1981) and over-reactiveness to sudden disturbances (Metz and Oosterlee 1980; Stolba and Wood-Gush 1980). Stereotypic behaviour mainly consists of the constant, compulsory repetition of certain motor patterns, resulting from a lack of general stimulation, or a lack of exercise. Redirected behaviour implies the fulfillment of behavioural needs on inadequate stimuli, and is often harmful or damaging to the animals, since parts of the body of mates often form the substitute for the original inanimate stimulus. Vacuum activity occurs when no appropriate stimulus is present at all, and the behaviour is performed "in the air," e.g., the air-chewing of sows in confinement. Over-reactiveness can be seen in, e.g., the alarm-reaction after sudden disturbances or the response to novel stimuli in a bare environment.

"In severely impoverished environments, arousal is generally increased,...due to an unsatisfied, strong motivation for certain activities" (Stolba and Wood-Gush 1980). By performing abnormal behaviour, the animal often "creates" its own stimulation, thereby reducing the increased arousal (Fox 1971; Vestergaard, 1981).

Again, as has been mentioned before, one can ask the question whether "abnormal behaviour actually is an advantage for the animal, since it reduces arousal" (Moss 1981b) but the answer must be "no" if we consider it from the perspective of the larger whole of an animal's nature and potentials.

A deprived animal, when placed in a rich environment, will overreact and indulge in a certain behaviour pattern (Wiepkema 1980). Even when an animal has been performing a certain behaviour on nonadequate objects e.g. bar-biting of sows, or "in the air" (vacuum-activities) it will immediately and strongly respond to adequate stimuli when these are given after the performance of displacement behaviour. This clearly indicates that an animal *does discriminate between adequate and nonadequate stimuli*, and that real satisfaction is not derived from adapted behaviour, otherwise the animal would not react so vigorously to adequate stimuli (Sambraus 1982; van Putten 1981; Stolba and Wood-Gush 1980). Sambraus mentions feeding and sexual behaviour as examples; sleep behaviour is furthermore added by Wiepkema. Stolba and Wood-Gush (1980) showed that the more bare the environment was, the stronger did piglets show the urge to explore new objects.

The fact that an animal has a telos, or intrinsic nature, implies that the fulfillment of its potential capacities matters fundamentally to it; every animal has a strong urge to be active and alert.

This is most clearly shown by some experiments which indicated that animals prefer to work for food, even if they do not have to. Markowitz (1982) describes how ostriches, who had learned to press key in order to obtain some peanuts as a reward, preferred to work in this way for their food instead of having it free. When a keeper accidentally dumped a whole bag of peanuts in their cage, they went over to the heap, sampled a few peanuts, and went back to their key to "earn" their peanuts. Wood-Gush (1973) mentions this phenomenon for chickens.

As others have repeatedly found, animals will typically work for food even when the same food is available free. This phenomenon "has been disquieting for some traditional learning theorists. After all, this illustrates how...superficial some of our explanations of animal behaviour are....We are emphatically confronted with the proposition that also animals like to do things, to see things change because of their efforts, to enjoy the pride of gathering their own food or drink, and to have some control over their lives. This is what behavioural enrichment is all about" (Markowitz 1982).

When an animal can fulfill its telos, and express its natural behaviour freely, it is generally recognized as being a contented or "happy" animal. Subjective experience, fulfillment and quality are inseparable aspects that come together in the behaviour of an animal.

What are the basic behavioural needs of animals, indicated by the concept of telos? Of course, this is basically different for each species, but attempts have been made to generalize some basic needs into behavioural categories.

BEHAVIOURAL NEEDS OF ANIMALS

In an attempt to determine behavioural needs of domestic animals, as well as those of laboratory animals, the question whether or not these animals are fundamentally different from their wild ancestors is a crucial one (Duncan 1981).

On a population level, adaptation is the result of changing gene frequencies (Beilharz 1982), caused by environmental pressures; a process called "natural selection." In the case of domestic species, another important factor has been selective breeding by man for certain desirable traits, such as docility and productivity.

It can be stated that those animals that have adapted their genotype continually to the demands created by man are very different from their wild ancestors (Beilharz 1982; Hughes 1980; Duncan 1981). An example of this might be the elimination of incubation and broody behaviour in the domestic chicken (Wood-Gush 1973; Craig 1982), although Brantas (1980) describes the frustration that occurs in hens that do not have a nest in which to lay their eggs. In the discussion after Brantas' presentation, it was remarked that the hens might have been frustrated because they had experienced laying in nests before. Whether behaviour is learned or not, it remains a fact that the animals respond adequately to stimuli which used to be a part of their ancestors' natural habitat.

Wood-Gush and Stolba (1982) report that pigs, kept in a "pig-park" with "a variety of environmental features, and a diversified social structure," show behaviour "that closely resembles behaviour described for the European wild boar." Boice (1981) in a review article of studies on captivity and feralization, states that "captivity and domestication do not necessarily produce behavioural degeneracies." As an example he mentions an experiment that showed that for albino

Norway rats, placed in an outdoor pen, "hundreds of generations of life in captivity have not altered the burrowing abilities of Norway rats." Systematic studies of the effects of feralization have shown that for a large number of species, animals placed in an outdoor pen resume their wild ways. Therefore, in order to understand the function of behavioural traits in domestic animals, and their importance for the animal, scientists need to study the wild ancestors of our domestic species thoroughly (Hartsock and Strickland, personal communication, 1982). Besides, domestication does not refer to today's intensive production systems. It is very unlikely that animals who always have been kept in extensive or semi-extensive conditions, have been able to adapt to the rapid changes of the past 20 years (Wood-Gush, as reported by Buchenauer, 1981).

So, on a population level, it is very likely that much of the potential for the full range of behaviour of wild ancestors is still present genetically, despite some selective, mostly physical changes. Baxter (1982/83) remarks that selective pressure on agricultural animals might even have strengthened original traits aimed at biological fitness rather than diminishing them. This would include traits like nesting behaviour. For zoo animals hardly any intentional selection takes place, and therefore their behavioural needs will resemble the needs of their wild conspecifics very much.

The following behavioural categories are considered to correspond with the most basic needs of animals:

Eating and drinking behaviour, especially search behaviour, is agreed upon by several authors to be crucially important (Fraser 1980; Sambraus 1981). A long list of abnormal and stereotypical behaviour related to this exists for many farm animal species (Sambraus 1981), indicating that the animal's internal drive to perform this behaviour is strong. He reports that when, for example, chickens are given their food in straw so that they have to search for it, they show a decreasing amount of abnormal feather-pecking. In zoos too, devices that are invented to make an animal work for his food rather than being fed at regular times, have caused drastic changes in formerly apathetic, inactive animals (Markowitz 1982).

Closely related to this are *explorative behaviour and locomotion*, considered almost as important as ingestive behaviour (Fraser 1980; Sambraus 1981). Stereotypic weaving of, e.g., polar bears and horses is interpreted to be evidence of lack of exercise and space to move, and disappears when more space is provided (Meijer-Holzapfel 1968; Fraser 1968). Daschbach *et al.* (1982/83) consider the importance of enough space for the locomotory behaviour of encaged monkeys (the slow lori, *Nycticebus concang*, in case), since too little space, especially if less than the so-called "flight-distance," can cause increased aggression, physical damage and resulting stress. (Flight distance refers to the linear distance between an animal and an animal of another species which is tolerated without fleeing.)

Exploratory behaviour is a strong drive, generally present in most animals, which serves to increase familiarity with the environment (Baxter 1982/83). Even when the possibility for locomotion is present, many abnormal adjustments appear when there is an absence of objects which are explorable. In pigs, for example, a well-known vice called tailbiting (which is a redirected activity) is considered to be directly related to a lack of exploratory possibilities, and causes significant economic losses (Sambraus 1981; Murphy 1978; Wiepkema 1982). Ekesbo, as reported by Duncan (1981) has shown that the incidence of trampled teats and clinical mastitis is higher when dairy cows are housed in small stalls without bedding. And these are only a few of the numerous examples of the damage that is done to animals physically and mentally by deprivation of adequate stimuli and the restriction of space.

The possibility of relating to the environment in a normal, healthy way is strongly represented by *play behaviour.* Especially for young animals, playing is of essential importance for their normal development, since it provides the possibility for a dialogue between the animal and its environment (Buchenauer 1981). Young animals develop their own ability for action through the interplay with the environment (Buchenauer 1981; Wood-Gush 1973); they acquire independence from the mother, learn to interact with peers (Jensen and Bobbit, cited by Fox, 1974) and develop motor control (Fraser 1980). By playing, the young animal gradually learns to be less dependent on its mother, and to control its environment on its own. "The entire basis for intelligence, for the acquisition of information, and for learning itself hinges upon early playful exploratory behaviour" (Fox 1974). Fraser (1980) further mentions *comfort activities* like grooming and nest-building, both of which are recognized as being of primary importance for the domestic chicken (Wood-Gush 1973; Hughes 1980), and the pig (Sambraus 1981); as well as sleeping and social behaviour.

As Fraser (1980) concludes, these needs seem formidable. But rather than being discouraged by the long list of behavioural needs, it might be important in this framework to summarize the discussion above by saying that most present animal-confinement systems, be it zoos, laboratories or intensive-production systems, have a great need for more "general stimulation," whatever stimuli this might imply.

Too little general stimulation, and a (fundamental) lack of the possibility for self-expression, deprive human beings and animals of a sense of fulfillment and satisfaction. In other words, a qualitatively poor environment leads to deprived, bored animals as a result (Murphy 1978).

BOREDOM AS A RESULT OF ENVIRONMENTAL DEPRIVATION

Considering environmental deprivation, it is meaningful to make a distinction between social environment and physical environment (Duncan 1981).

Clearly, for social animals the social environment is of crucial importance. All agricultural domestic animals are social species, which means that they normally live in groups with an organized social structure (Duncan 1981). Most laboratory animals such as mice, rats, dogs and monkeys are social animals, too. Duncan mentions and discusses several possible kinds of social deprivation: prevention of the formation of a parent-offspring bond, early weaning, the keeping of animals in single-age or single-sex groups, and isolation. Some effects of social deprivation are a higher mortality, increased aggression, displacement behaviour (e.g., calves, lambs and piglets who are weaned early suck each other, or perform vacuum-sucking behaviour); distorted behaviour (such as isolated cockerels chasing their own tails), physiological effects like a high incidence of arteriosclerosis (Duncan 1981) and "learned" helplessness (Fox 1983a).

However, since a more common problem in farms is overcrowding, rather than social deprivation (Murphy 1978), it is mainly the impoverished *physical* environment that makes people question animal-keeping systems like zoos, laboratories and intensive production units. The so-called "barren environment" is referred to by many authors in their discussion of animal welfare (Hughes 1980; van Putten 1982b; Wood-Gush 1973; Duncan 1981; Buchenauer 1981; Brantas 1975). "What could be more unhealthy than an unresponsive environment?" Markowitz (1982) asks in his book about behavioural enrichment in zoos. He reports on the beneficial effect that environmental enrichment had on the performance of species-specific behaviour of polar bears: reduced stereotypic activity, greatly improved physical health (not in the least because they stopped begging for junk-food from zoo visitors), and reduced aggressive behaviour of males towards newborns. All too familiar is the stereotypic behaviour of caged zoo animals, from canaries, foxes, coyotes, bears, etc., to great apes. The latter are also known to eat their own vomit and faeces (Fox 1971).

For laboratory animals, nervous anorexia, coprophagia (eating of faeces), polyphagia and polydipsia (eating and drinking too much), as well as asocial, stereotypic and aggressive behaviour can be results of social and environmental deprivation (Fox 1974).

A related area of concern is the lack of general stimulation for dogs and cats in shelters. Isolation and understimulation can cause hysterical, high-pitched barking, abnormal behaviour such as a dog chasing his own tail, and a general appearance of nonalertness: dull coats and eyes. This can be improved by providing toys such as sticks, balls and blankets. But for animals used to being so close to human beings, the most important need they have is human contact. All other needs such as exercise, play etc., are dependent on the presence or absence of human attention. To have a relationship with human beings has become the most important aspect of the nature of a dog; far more so than for a cat (Wright, personal communication, 1982). However, even for piglets the presence of two human caretakers can make a difference of 5 kilograms growth per pig per 6 weeks! (Hammer 1980).

In Part II, the problem of environmental deprivation in agricultural animals will be discussed more elaborately. Many scientists use the term "boredom" with or without quotes, in talking about the subjective experience of animals in a deprived environment (Wood-Gush 1973, 1981; Murphy 1978; Duncan 1981; Griffin 1981b; Humphrey 1981; Kiley-Worthington 1981; Vestergaard 1981). This phenomenon can be explained biologically in terms of "a motivational state which drives the animal to increase its overall sensory input" (Murphy 1978; see also Griffin 1981b).

But before it can be accepted that animals can be bored, there are some questions that have to be considered first, according to several authors. Can one apply a concept like boredom to "an animal as primitive as a fowl, particularly if its behaviour is largely governed by releasers?" (Wood-Gush 1973). "Does it matter to an animal whether the necessary stimulation comes from the environment directly or whether from themselves by performing a stereotypy in a non-stimulating environment?' (Murphy 1978). Is boredom a term which applies only to humans, as Duncan (1981) says, and which does *not* refer to an equivalent mental experience in animals (Murphy 1978; Humphrey 1981)?

Although several authors raise these questions, most of them go no further than to offer a few speculatory lines. Griffin (1981b) suggests that "since laboratory rodents will run several kilometers every night in an exercise wheel, while wild conspecifics never seem to go more than 100 m. from their nest, the laboratory animal might be bored." Some people say, however, that despite all the evidence that animals do prefer to respond to external stimuli when these are present, this still does not answer the question whether animals miss what they do not know (Ewbank 1981), or whether they actually suffer in the absence of stimuli (Wood-Gush 1973). Because intuitively, that seems to be what boredom implies: *missing stimuli that should be there but are not.*

The presence of stereotypies in zoos and laboratory animals, and all domestic species, however, strongly suggests that an animal does miss general stimulation, otherwise it would not develop these highly repetitive, unnatural behaviour patterns to stimulate itself, nor would it engage in all kinds of harmful and physically injurious displacement activities. This is where the second question comes in: does it matter to the animal *how* it satisfies its need for stimulation; do animals have a sense of "quality of life" as suggested by Murphy (1978).

From a reductionist point of view, there might be no decisive answer to this question. Subjective experience is considered to be a secondarily derived factor in reductionistic explanatory models. A fundamental way of taking subjective experience seriously, as a central feature of life, requires a shift of observational perspective (or "*gestalt-shift*").

From such a perspective we see behaviour not solely as a means towards a reproductive end. Baxter's (1982/83) statement that behaviour is "one way of accommodating requirements, and not the requirement itself" is direct evidence of an approach which reduces the animal to a functional mechanism. In this approach boredom could not exist as long as the desired production were guaranteed. A shift from quantity to quality does imply that behaviour is seen as the requirement itself.

In this framework *an animal can be said to be bored when it has to adapt to its environment in an abnormal way, indicative of understimulation, in order to maintain its sense of selfhood.* The continuity between man and animal, and the evidence for feeling and awareness in animals (see Section I, *The Question of Animal Awareness*, in this volume) imply that boredom is a direct subjective experience of an animal.

It is not always easy to distinguish "boredom" from "frustration." Boredom can give rise to frustration, e.g. when a sow tries to break away from its ties to build a nest, or when aggression in battery cage hens increases as a result of deprivation of nesting boxes for laying-behaviour. An aggressive bird can hardly be called a bored one, yet it is important to realize the close link between the two phenomena. Boredom could be regarded as a qualitative description of the psychological state that gives rise to general frustration.

An advanced form of boredom is the phenomenon of helplessness, elaborately described by Seligman (1975) for human beings, and by Fox (1983a) for animals. After a prolonged time of lack of control and predictability over the environment, animals "give up" trying to express themselves and become apathetic. Van Putten describes this for tethered sows: the sow sits, lets its head hang down and has its eyes nearly closed. This has been referred to as "mourning" behaviour (van Putten 1982b; see also Fox 1983a). In laboratory animals it is often present as a result of experiments, and the animal's inability to control its life (Fox 1982). Helplessness is characterized by the general refusal to respond, even to novel stimuli, or damage being done to its own body; these traits distinguish helplessness clearly from habituation (Fox 1983a). Further effects are decreased learning ability, immunosuppression, loss of weight and appetite, norepinephrine depletion and increased cholinergic activity (Fox 1983a).

Helplessness is the pathological mental state arising from the animal's conviction that, whatever it does, it cannot have any real control over its environment. It believes (or has learned) that responding is useless, since there will be no reinforcement to the response (Seligman 1975). If lack of natural stimuli can produce such a pathological state, equivalent to mental illness and depression in humans, then surely it matters to an animal that it be provided with an environment that gives it the chance to be a mentally and physically healthy animal, rather than a bored or helpless one.

THE SCIENTIFIC ACCESSIBILITY OF BOREDOM

Although there have been no attempts to conduct systematic research about the phenomenon of boredom, methods to do so might be indicated.

Discussing possible parameters for the observation of boredom, it is helpful to realize that boredom is a relative as well as an absolute phenomenon. It is relative in the sense that animals perform a greater variety of behaviour patterns in a more stimulating environment, and therefore any environment can be said to be boring in comparison to a richer environment. A rich environment can give us an idea of the behavioural potential of different animal species, and may serve in this way as a frame of reference for the evaluation of understimulating environments, and for the interpretation of the abnormal behaviour occurring in them. Boredom is an absolute phenomenon so far as lack of stimulation becomes apparent in abnormal behaviour patterns.

For adequate observations of an environment that is suspected to be boring, the following conditions seem to be essential:

1. A thorough knowledge of the species-specific behaviour and its development in a rich, stimulating environment, whether it be wild or domestic.
2. Observations of animal behaviour over long periods of time, preferably 24 hours, or 12 hours a day. The occurrence of different behaviour patterns can be evaluated best in this way, since boredom is a concept related to time.
3. The presence of the observer must be concealed, or it must be certain that this does not influence the behaviour of the animals

in any way. In relation to boredom this is especially important since human presence is itself a stimulation which might temporarily obscure evidence of boredom.

The following criteria for boredom are proposed:

1. Stereotypic movements.
2. Redirected activity which occurs systematically towards inadequate stimuli.
3. Vacuum behaviour.
4. General apathy and immobility over longer periods, accompanied by an inalert expression in the eyes, if possible to observe. This includes longer periods of sitting and standing.

The first three behaviours are evidence of the fact that an animal is still trying to cope with a lack of stimulation. The fourth, advanced state of boredom indicates the impossibility for the animal to express itself; it has more or less given up trying to adapt to the situation.

The presence of any one of these behaviours is a direct indication of the fact that the environment is inadequate for the behavioural needs of an animal. It is generally agreed that understimulation is the main cause for the behaviour patterns which are proposed as indicators of boredom. Everyone who spends a short time in a particular intensive production system can observe the presence of stereotypic behaviour, vacuum activities or redirected activities such as forms of cannibalism. These are all *qualitative* indicators that the environment is a boring one to which the animals have to adapt in an abnormal way. As was said before, larger periods of observation are desirable for a more detailed scientific description of the situation. However, it is questionable whether at present this is really necessary. Much is known already about the occurrence of abnormal behaviour in farm animals, enough to indicate the actual need for environmental enrichment in intensive systems.

Accepting that boredom is an adverse state, it can be regarded as a form of stress for the animal. Stress is a phenomenon that has mainly been studied in terms of internal processes. That is, what are the effects of external stressors on homeostasis, which is the regulation of the internal environment to maintain an internal equilibrium. In order to gain insight into the way boredom acts as a stressor on an animal, a general theoretical framework of stress will be discussed. Central questions in the development of such a framework appear to be "what is normal?" and "is the maintenance of homeostasis a good criterion for the absence of stress?" Secondly, "what are the best parameters for abnormal, stressful states?" As will become clear, the last question concentrates on the usefulness of behavioural versus physiological parameters.

BOREDOM AS A STRESSOR

Within the difficult and vague field of stress research, the concept of a General Adaptation Syndrome (GAS), as developed by Hans Selye was a major breakthrough (Moss 1981a; Friend 1980; Ewbank 1973). One of the important aspects of his work was his distinction between "stressors" and "stress response," the first referring to adverse or noxious stimuli, the latter to the mechanisms by which an animal resists the effects of adverse stimuli (Ewbank 1973; Moss 1981a). He defined stress as a specific syndrome in a biological system, consisting of all nonspecific responses to a stressor.

Although Selye's work is still very influential, Fraser, Ritchie and Fraser (1975) have pointed out that the concept might be too simple. First, specific stressors may not only generate nonspecific responses but very specific ones as well (Siegèl 1980; Dantzer & Morméde 1981), depending on the nature of the stressor. Second, while overstimulation might cause a certain (general) reaction, it has become clear that animals can be understimulated as well, which might also cause a physiological reaction. In terms of the response of the animal, one could speak of "understress," "stress" and "overstress" in this context, thereby indicating that "stress" in itself is not adverse, but that only extreme effects are deleterious to the animal (Ewbank 1973; Freeman 1978).

This immediately raises the question whether it is possible to determine a "normal" baseline of stress in order to see which stressors are "beneficial" (building up biological fitness) and which are adverse (Fraser, Ritchie and Fraser 1975; Freeman 1976; Perry 1973). A study on the variance in corticosteroid levels during egg-laying in hens (Beuving 1980) showed also, however, that changes in normal behaviour correspond to variations in hormone concentration. This makes it very hard to interpret any response of the adrenal glands as adverse or normal. In fact, an animal is never in a static state, but always acting and reacting to external and internal stimuli, in order to maintain a state of internal, physiological homeostasis (Ewbank 1973).

This state of homeostasis is widely regarded as the "normal" state. "The psychological setpoint at which there is no effect on welfare, represents the homeostatic setpoint" (Baxter 1982/83). Behaviour, in this context, is regarded as the means by which an animal maintains homeostasis and adapts to the environment (Wiepkema 1982; Buré 1981a).

If the pressure of certain stimuli rises, however, and it becomes harder for an animal to maintain a homeostatic equilibrium, the internal stress-response leads to a stage which is referred to as "the resistance stage," a concept introduced by Selye (Fraser, Ritchie and

Fraser 1975). If the stressors in the environment are too severe, or are present too long, the stress-response proceeds into the so-called "exhaustion stage" which will result in death, if nothing is done (Freeman 1978; McBride 1979).

It is now widely believed that *adaptation* to a stressful situation (a stressor) *eliminates* that event from being a stressor (Friend 1980 referring to Mobey), which implies that only when an animal's physiological state is in the stage of exhaustion, can it truly be called stressed in its adverse meaning (McBride 1979; Perry 1973). A very practical aspect of accepting this concept of stress is that in domestic situations, most animals are slaughtered before they could reach the exhaustion stage, and therefore it is hard to determine whether some stimuli should be classified as highly stressful or not (McBride 1979; Freeman 1975). Furthermore, the psychophysiological costs of adaptation, which may lower the animal's ability to cope with additional stressors, need to be considered when it is believed that an animal has actually adapted to a given set of stressors.

In the model of stress outlined above, "normal" as a standard for an acceptable level of stress-response can be replaced by "adapted" (Bessei 1980), and is represented by a homeostatic state.

Several authors agree upon the fact that stress primarily must be determined by means of physiological parameters, since homeostasis is a physiological phenomenon (Freeman 1976; McBride 1979; Friend 1980). "...It is quite clear that evidence will come from physiologists and not ethologists. It is they who must face the problems of measurement and definition" (McBride 1979). If, after the initial acute physiological response to adverse stimuli, physiological changes *remain*, it might well mean that the situation has become too severe and that the animal cannot adapt through its behaviour. This is the worst kind of stress, leading to death. If the initial physiological response disappears after a while because of behavioural adaptation, then the developed homeostatic state is not recognized as stressful according to the framework presented above. In other words, a decrease of physiological deviation is directly correlated to a decrease of stress. Abnormal behaviour has been reported to cause a decrease in corticosteroid reaction (Dantzer 1981; Buré 1981b; Dantzer and Mormède 1981), and therefore might be regarded not as a sign of stress, but as *a means towards decreasing stress* (Wiepkema 1982; Dantzer and Mormède 1981).

It must be questioned whether it is appropriate to consider homeostasis as a standard of what is "normal" in this respect, since *the price that animals have to pay in order to be able to adapt* is completely left out of account. And the distortion of the intrinsic nature of an animal, caused by the performance of abnormal behaviour, is a high price indeed.

As Fraser, Ritchie and Fraser (1975) pointed out, from a veterinarian, animal-centered point of view, the *quality of the process* of coping is as important as the final result. Referring to "the perennial disagreement" about the question whether behavioural disruptions could by themselves be regarded as symptoms of stress, without physiological confirmation, they state that this is justified, since "a system of husbandry is clearly in need of improvement if adverse consequences are prevented only by gross changes in either behaviour *or* physiology" (emphasis added).

To understand the role behavioural and physiological factors play it is important not just to understand the relationship between behaviour and physiology, but to understand first of all the relationship of *each* of them with the nature, or beingness of the animal.

First of all, it is possible that there are as yet unknown physiological indicators, other than adrenocortical hormones, which do correlate with emotional behaviour. Heart-rate, cardiac output or skin-resistence (Baldwin and Stephens 1971) or other neurohormonal systems (Dantzer and Mormède 1981) have been mentioned as possibilities. In this case behaviour and physiology would both refer to the same state of being of the animal. The suggestion that there also might be a fundamental difference regarding their function for the animal is elucidated by Seligman (1975), in his book *Helplessness*. Since helplessness is an advanced form of boredom, as was described earlier, Seligman's remarks apply very well to the study of boredom. After discussing several experiments, he concludes that the neurotransmitter norepinephrine (NE) level appears to be a very important physiological parameter for a feeling of control over the environment in humans and animals. However, he goes on, "NE-depletion alone cannot account for many of the facts that the cognitive theory predicts, since NE-depletion seems to be neither necessary nor sufficient to produce learned helplessness...The difference between escapability and inescapability is not physical; *it is information that can only be processed cognitively.*" The way in which this information is processed in a particular situation depends on the *behavioural possibilities* the animal has for controlling its environment (e.g. to escape or not). Cognition and emotion are inseparable (Seligman 1975) and so cognition, emotion and behavioural possibilities are linked on the same level of integration, namely the highest one possible, and equivalent to the concepts of "nature," "telos" or "beingness." Considering Seligman's results it can be concluded that stress in general and boredom in particular *are best assessed by behavioral parameters*, rather than by physiological ones. The idea that physiology is a form of behaviour as well (Wiepkema, personal communication 1982) obscures the presence of a qualitative difference between the two: behaviour has to do with the "whole" integrated animal, whereas physiology reflects the interaction of the various (unconscious) parts. Physiological factors cannot be weighed on the same scale as behavioural ones, though they can certainly be useful indicators.*

With the definition of stress given by Fraser, Ritchie and Fraser (1975), there is room for the considerations discussed above: "an abnormal or extreme adjustments in its behaviour or physiology, in order to cope with adverse aspects of its environment and management."

So far we have argued that homeostasis is not an adequate criterion for "normal," since it ignores the price an animal has to pay for its adaptation. It was also argued that behaviour as a parameter for stressful states is, qualitatively speaking, the most appropriate one. This shift in emphasis might make it easier to determine what is "normal" when we have to speak of "abnormal or extreme adjustments." "Extreme" and "abnormal" in a behavioural context do not refer to a numerical scale anymore as would be the case with physiological parameters, but to a qualitative change in behavioural adjustment. Redirected activity like tail-biting for example can then be regarded as an indicator of stress, since it is a form of abnormal behaviour.

Rather then speaking of understress, stress and overstress, *abnormal adjustments could be indicated by using the terms "stress" and "distress;"* distress being caused by understimulation, and stress by overstimulation. In this way "normal" refers to a certain level of "healthy" stimulation by specific stimuli (van Putten 1981), and not to a normal level of "stress." It is true that animals need a certain amount of stimulating "pressure" from the environment to develop their "fitness," their flexible response to changing conditions. But if the terms "understress" and "overstress" were used as Ewbank (1973) proposed, thereby accepting the "normality" of stress, or even calling it beneficial (Ewbank 1973), the adverse quality of the term "stress" would be very much diminished and thereby lose most of its meaning.

Boredom, in the framework developed above, can be characterized as a form of distress, resulting from chronic understimulation. Important criteria are the different forms of abnormal behaviour, mentioned in the previous paragraph. In physiology, hardly any relevant research about the effects of understimulation has been done; a few relevant experiments will be discussed shortly. It seems important to consider

*Psychological-cognitive and emotional factors can be more potent in producing physiological changes such as increased production of natural opiates than physical trauma per se (Miczek, K.A. et al. 1982. *Science* 215:1520–1522)—Ed.

that the physiological reaction towards understimulation might be (fundamentally) different from the reaction to overstimulation, which is aimed at a homeostatic equilibrium.

CONSEQUENCES FOR THE FIELD OF ANIMAL WELFARE

In order to make it possible for the natural sciences to study animal well-being, an operational definition of "well-being" is necessary. The definition given by Lorz (1979) has been widely accepted as useful in this context: "welfare implies a state of harmony, both physical and psychological, of the animal with itself and with its environment. Health and normal behaviour are usually indicators for well-being. They presuppose a life-course which is species-specific, and which does justice to species-specific behaviour."

As can be seen from the previous paragraphs boredom represents a serious impairment of well-being as defined above since it implies a fundamental lack of behavioural possibilities for an animal. Yet in a larger context, so it is argued by many, this kind of suffering is only relative. In nature, animals experience all kinds of other, harmful and adverse conditions, such as bad weather, lack of food and the pressure of predators. These are eliminated in intensive farm systems, where the basic existence of an animal is guaranteed. How can we ever weigh these different elements on an overall scale of well-being?

The argument implies that an ideal situation is not possible, and therefore the present husbandry system might give an animal a different environment from its natural one, but not necessarily a worse one. However, this line of thought leaves out the fact that we as humans have consciously taken responsibility for the lives and well-being of our farm animals. Natural conditions for wild animals are beyond human responsibility, but it lies fully within our power to provide farm animals with whatever they need, "and there can be no justification for continuation of the conditions once severe strain has been diagnosed" (McBride 1979). Not providing animals with the opportunity to express their behavioural needs is therefore a conscious choice, dependent upon our own moral and economic standards. Only from a dualistic perspective can one compare natural and confinement conditions as if they were two "objective" situations. From an involved perspective, it is clear that however thoroughly we study needs and adaptive capacities of animals, in the end it remains a subjective choice whether we realize certain options for the animal or not; whether we force an animal to adapt, or give it room to express its basic behavioural drives. "Potentiality is an unseen reality," and as long as we know that we could give an animal more stimulation, we will have to find good reasons not to give it, however great the animal's adaptive capacities.

Another option we have in the conflict present in farms, laboratories and zoos between the animal's needs and its actual environment, is not to adjust the environment to the animal, but the animal to the environment. By altering its genetic make-up fundamentally through selection and genetic manipulation, we could "create" animals whose needs can be fulfilled in a man-made, economically oriented environment. By selecting animals "that are less aware of their environment and so less likely to be distressed by it" (Duncan 1973), general animal welfare could be "improved" according to several authors (Craig 1982; Fauré 1980; Beilharz 1982). Raymond (1980) rejects this idea, however, not on ethical grounds but for the practical reason that it takes a very long time; in the meantime our economic needs or ethical framework might change, and then it would be hard to reverse the process. Adjusting the environment to the animal is more efficient on a short-term basis and more flexible. But apart from the practical objections, one can have serious ethical objections. Changing animals in this way is again one step further on the road of the manipulation of life and the acquisition of power over the world. I do not see this as a desirable direction, and I think we would harm ourselves as much as the animals by alienating ourselves in this way from natural life.

Boredom is a serious problem in present husbandry systems. In the next section evidence for this statement will be provided, and the importance of boredom in relation to other parameters of well-being will be discussed.

PART II

BOREDOM IN AGRICULTURAL PRODUCTION SYSTEMS

We have noted earlier that very little serious research about animal boredom has been performed. But work on closely related subjects such as housing systems and stereotypic behaviour is very relevant to our understanding of boredom.

In the field of farm animal welfare, most research on environmental deprivation seems to be concentrated on battery cage chickens and on sows and their litters kept in close confinement. Cows appear to have much less need for external stimulation. This may be due to their rumination process, which provides self-stimulation via chewing of the cud and grooming, and thus "boredom and aggression are reduced in establishing groups of cattle" (Albright 1982). Yet in veal calves boredom might be considered a serious problem. Because of isolation and lack of opportunity to fulfill their needs, calves lick and suck themselves, other calves, walls and inanimate objects. Health problems are often the result (Albright 1982).

A general description of present housing systems of pigs and chickens will now be given, and behavioural and physiological evidence of boredom in these systems presented. The effect that boredom has on other welfare criteria such as productivity, reproductivity, disease susceptibility, etc., will be discussed and a general evaluation of boredom as an indicator of welfare closes this section.

HOUSING SYSTEMS

The housing systems of chickens and sows have changed dramatically since the 1930's (Sainsbury 1978) and 1950's (van Putten 1982a). Our improved technological ability to develop a completely artificially controlled microclimate (Sainsbury 1978), the rapidly growing monopoly of the animal-feed industry (van Putten 1982a), the role of genetic science in the selection for productive animals, along with the increasing cost of land and labour, have worked together to press farmers to move the animals from outside yards to increasingly restricted environments, "where technical demands were given a higher priority than the animal's basic needs" (Ekesbo 1981a). As a result "commercial egglayers" are housed mostly in multibird cages with the birds kept in groups of 3 to 5 with considerable restriction of movements (Sainsbury 1978).

Sows are usually kept in individual pens and are tethered, preventing social contact with other sows. The floor is bare; oestrus is usually induced with hormones (because spontaneous oestrus disappears in the absence of social contact), and piglets are weaned at ever earlier ages (Lean 1978).

BEHAVIOURAL EVIDENCE FOR BOREDOM IN PIGS AND CHICKENS

Sows and piglets

"The type of pigs most affected by the extreme changes in housing systems are sows" (Buchenauer 1981). Tethering or restraint deprives them of their natural tendency to be active and inquisitive, and the lives of sows have become "extremely dull" (van Putten 1982b); their great need to explore the environment is reflected in their continuous use (given the opportunity) of their very sensitive noses (Hartsock, personal communication, 1982). In an article on sow health and housing Ekesbo (1981a) reports that tied sows are significantly less active during daytime than loose sows (respectively 32% versus 59%). During this active time the loose sows carried out 12 different behaviour patterns with straw while for the tied sows, only two or three behaviour patterns involving straw were observed. Furthermore, Ekesbo (1981a) also notes that pig breeders have always given their animals separate areas for feeding, defecating and lying. Recent investigations have shown that loose sows divide their time in these three areas accompanied by 1216 social interactions, with 12 different patterns of behaviour. Tied sows only performed 236 interactions, while three patterns were completely absent.

Daelemans (1981) also argues that loose sows have a chance to move between separate areas for drinking and eating, thereby being able to gratify their apparently highly motivated need for exercise (Ekesbo 1981a). Baxter (1981) adds nest building to the list of behavioural needs. Restrained sows can be observed trying to break away before farrowing, because of their high motivation to move around and arrange a nesting area (van Putten 1982b; Buchenauer 1981; Vestergaard 1981).

Restrained sows demonstrate a high incidence of abnormal behaviour, which can be as much as 17.5% of the whole range of behaviour patterns (Buchenauer 1981). Stereotypical behaviour such as "weaving;" redirected activity such as "bar-biting," licking bars, trough floor and chain; "play-drinking," and vacuum behaviour such as "teethgrinding," "air-chewing," "tongue rolling" and rooting; and a general restlessness, are strong evidence of frustration due to lack of adequate stimuli (Ekesbo 1981a; Vestergaard 1981; Sambraus 1981; van Putten 1982b; Buchenauer 1981). Other indicators are the long periods, up to six hours, of "sitting," which has been attributed to significant drowsiness (Buchenauer 1981). Vestergaard (1981), Sambraus (1981) and Fraser (1968) report observations of sows sitting with their heads hanging down, or pressed against the stall divisions. Standing, which occurs for long periods, may be regarded as a conflict between the desire for activity and the impossibility to achieve it (Buchenauer 1981).

The absence of straw also appears to be a significant deprivation. The effect of its presence or absence is discussed by many authors (Ekesbo 1981a; Vestergaard 1981; Sambraus 1981). Vestergaard (1981) reports in fact that oral and other stereotypies (such as weaving, vacuum-chewing, bar-biting) were reduced by loose straw. He found that such abnormal behaviour would increase within a few days after the removal of straw and decrease as soon as straw was present. This suggests that stereotypic behaviour might not be a remnant, left over from adaptation to some adverse situation in the past (Wiepkema 1982), but an immediate response to the adequacy of the environment. At the same time, straw could be used as nest building material (van Putten 1982b).

Piglets are never restrained, but the effect of the absence or presence of straw on their behaviour has been reported in several studies. When straw is present, rooting and chewing are more common, and other patterns such as nest building behaviour and play with the straw are elicited (Troxler 1980; van Putten and Dammers 1976). When straw is absent, redirected exploratory behaviour such as nibbling on other piglets and inanimate objects occurs (Troxler 1980; van Putten and Dammers 1976; Buchenauer 1981). Tail-biting is reported to be positively correlated with the absence of straw, since the provision of straw reduces this behaviour (Sambraus 1981; Buchenauer 1981; Koomans 1981). Therefore tail-biting might be a sign of boredom (Ewbank 1981; Bareham and Vestergaard 1981). In the straw barn, playing and fighting occur more than in cages (Bure 1981a), so straw in pig pens provides play material and reduces boredom (Bareham and Vestergaard 1981). "By enriching even a small environment, ...their reactivity towards unfamiliar stimuli drops dramatically, and approaches the low intensity and short duration seen under semi-natural condition" (Stolba and Wood-Gush 1980).

The long list of stereotypic and conflict behaviour, related to exploratory behaviour, feeding behaviour and locomotion in a richer environment where the sows are not restrained, provides evidence that boredom is a real problem for pigs in modern confinement systems without straw or some other substance to stimulate various natural behaviours.

CHICKENS IN BATTERY CAGES

The chicken is a very different animal and is also considered to be more primitive than a pig (Duncan 1981). Nevertheless, "deprivation of external stimuli is a factor to be considered even in an animal as phylogenetically primitive as a fowl" (Wood-Gush 1973).

Compared to deep litter pens, battery cages restrict behavioural patterns such as turning, dust-bathing, ground-pecking, wing-flapping, movement flapping and general locomotion (Bareham 1972, 1976; Duncan 1979; Hughes 1978). Furthermore, the absence of litter and nest boxes makes dust-bathing and nesting behaviour impossible.

As was observed for pigs above, the restriction of several behavioural possibilities is accompanied by a range of abnormal behaviour patterns, like stereotypic movements and redirected activities. The most prevalent abnormalities are feather-pecking, as a form of cannibalism, stereotypic pacing, stereotypic headflicking, displacement preening and vacuum dust-bathing.

"The most important factor contributing to feather-pecking is the absence of litter" (Duncan 1978). This is supported by experiments conducted by Bareham (1976). Hughes (1978) suggests that rather than being a result of boredom, feather-pecking is a substitute for ground-pecking. However, redirected activities *are* regarded as signs of boredom since they indicate the lack of stimuli. Feather-pecking can be compared to tail-biting in pigs: one animal, probably genetically disposed, starts the vice, and the others "learn" it from a few initiators (Duncan 1978; Sambraus 1981). Sambraus also states that, if chickens are fed on the ground instead of a trough, this reduces feather-pecking.

Stereotypic pacing is usually regarded as a sign of frustration due to the impossibility of performing nest building behaviour in a battery cage (Hughes 1978; Duncan 1978; Bareham 1976; Brantas 1980; Wood-Gush 1973; Fölsch 1980). Experimentally frustrated hens, in fact, do exhibit stereotypic pacing (Duncan 1978).

Head-flicking in laying hens described by Bareham (1972) can be compared to an equivalent sort of head turn in zoo animals when they are engaged in stereotypic pacing (Bareham 1972; Fox 1971). Its occurrence can be attributed to a monotonous environment with a restriction of external stimuli. This behaviour can be seen as the animal's attempt to increase its sensory input (Bareham 1972; Duncan 1981). Compensatory feeding behaviour, where chickens play with their food for long periods, without a higher intake of food, can be regarded as a compensation for other behaviour which has become impossible. A similar phenomenon occurs in pigs. Excessive preening can likewise be interpreted as a sign of "mild frustration" in the form of compensatory activity (Bareham 1976; Duncan 1979). The occurrence of vacuum dust-bathing indicates the innate need for a hen to perform this behaviour (Hughes 1980; Vestergaard 1981). The same is true of the need for wing-flapping and body/wing shaking, which may accumulate as well during deprivation (Vestergaard 1981).

Aggression might be considered as a sign of frustration due to deprivation, since it can be reduced by providing hens with a nest box (Vestergaard 1981). Vestergaard furthermore states that this indicates that "the birds really do miss those things."

From the evidence presented above, it can be concluded that boredom, as defined earlier, is a concept applicable to the chicken as well. The fact that they miss exploration-eliciting stimuli, and stimuli that facilitate other natural behaviour, can be inferred from the presence of many abnormal behaviour patterns, and from experiments that have shown that chickens prefer to work for their food rather than have it available freely (Wood-Gush 1973).

PHYSIOLOGICAL INDICATORS OF BOREDOM

Although it was suggested that stress, and distress due to understimulation, are detected mainly through behavioural phenomena, this does not mean that there are no physiological indicators. However, hardly any direct research into physiological responses to understimulation has yet been done. It is known from several experiments (Dantzer and Mormède 1981; Wiepkema 1982) that deprivation can originally lead to rise of plasma corticosteroid levels. But stereotypic behaviour such as chain-nibbling in pigs during food deprivation reduces the hormone levels considerably (Dantzer and Mormède 1981). As a result of these experiments it was concluded that circulating ACTH and corticosteroid levels are not sensitive to chronic stress (which boredom is considered to be). However, Barnett, Hemsworth, and Hand (1982/83) do refer to corticosteroid levels as parameters for chronic stress, based on experiments about the effect of handling pigs. Corticosteroids might be sensitive to chronic stress, therefore, but not to chronic *distress*. This is supported by the fact that none of the three studies done so far on understimulation in chickens indicates any difference between battery cages and deep litter pens in adrenal activity (Freeman 1978). One can speculate that there may be physiological indicators that correlate with understimulation, e.g. the neurotransmitter norepinephrine (Seligman 1975).

THE EFFECT OF BOREDOM ON PHYSICAL CHARACTERISTICS OF AN ANIMAL

Production

A bored pig is a slower growing pig, and "time is money" (Jesse, *Wall Street Journal*-11/1982). Jesse reported that a group of pigs, moved around to other, identical pens twice before slaughter, gained 1 pound more per pig per week than a control group. More stimulation, and a different view of the other pigs around them, are given as the explanation for this. Similar results were found by Koomans (1981): fattening pigs housed in an open front piggery with straw had a significantly higher average daily gain, and higher average back fat, than those without straw. The average food conversion was the same, which indicates that the animals ate more per day. This was also noted by

Jesse who stated of his pigs that "they felt better and ate better." As tail-biting may result in condemnation to death at the abbatoir, straw given to prevent tail-biting can minimize production loss in an indirect way (Bareham and Vestergaard 1981).

In chicken farming both better and worse production have been observed in pens compared to cages (Bareham 1972). The occurrence of cannibalism and extreme flightiness does decrease egg production (Craig 1982), but how this correlates with housing in cages or pens is not clear. There are many different factors at work, and a definitive experiment has not yet been carried out.

Reproduction

The adverse effects of restraint on sows are indicated by a number of results. First, sows come into heat earlier in a free-range environment, the main reason being the social stimulation from other sows (van Putten 1982a), but also because piglets suckle less. The constant suckling in intensive systems retards oestrus (Stolba 1982). In an indirect way, restraint, and thereby the prevention of nesting behaviour, affects reproduction: the resulting stress can cause inflammation of udder and uterus, and lactation becomes impossible. This syndrome is especially prevalent in gilts. Also, indications have been found that restraint at farrowing increases the incidence of still births, mummified piglets and piglets with splaylegs (Baxter 1981; Ekesbo 1981a).

Disease—susceptibility

An increase in the frequency of disease in sows correlates with the increased restraint of sows in confinement systems. It is not unusual that continuous medication is needed to prevent disease, and this is a poor way of maintaining the animal's health compared to changing the environment (Ekesbo 1981a; Buchenauer 1981). Concerning the direct correlation between exploratory behaviour and disease, different studies have shown that there is a significantly higher incidence of Salmonella (diarrhea) infection in herds with no straw (Metz and Oosterlee 1980; Ekesbo 1981b), although rationally the opposite might be expected because straw may be seen as a good medium for building up an infection fast (Truyen 1981). Backström's studies of environmental factors showed that general health was better in pens with straw compared to other beddings, and much better than in pens with no bedding (Ekesbo 1981a).

In this same line Metz and Oosterlee (1980) found a lower antibody level and therefore a greater disease susceptibility, of tethered sows in pens without straw, compared with free sows in pens with straw. Total morbidity, and also the occurrence of the mastitis syndrome (agalactia toxemia) was shown to be much higher for tethered sows; the litters of tethered sows in a small pen had a higher total morbidity than litters of free sows in large pens (Ekesbo 1981a).

For sows and piglets it seems there is a direct correlation between disease susceptibility and restraint and the absence of straw, which are considered to be the two conditions which are very likely to cause boredom. Besides diarrhea and mastitis, infectious pneumonia is a frequently occurring and highly damaging illness in pig operations.

For fowl, experimental work has been done on the effect of stress on disease susceptibility (Freeman 1976; Siegel 1980). How these results apply to the different aspects of battery cage life is not clear; only the effects of social stress as a result of reduced space have been examined (Siegel 1980) and were found to cause decreased antibody levels and greater susceptibility to viral diseases such as New Castle disease, Marek's disease, hemorrhagic enteritis, and Salmonella infection. (However, resistance to bacterial infection seemed to be increased.) Most of these stress factors are coupled with a rise in corticosteroid levels (Freeman 1976), but Freeman also reports that antibody production can be shown "to be impaired by stressors which do not even evoke a rise in plasma corticosterone. If more research would be done in this field, it might be speculated that lack of stimulation, and resulting boredom and frustration, can be forms of non-corticosteroid mediated chronic stress that affect antibody production."

PHYSICAL INJURY

The most obvious examples of physical injury as a result of boredom are the vices of tail-biting in pigs and feather-pecking in laying hens. These are countered by debeaking hens and cutting the tails of newly born piglets. From a welfare point this is unacceptable, certainly for the hen, since the beak is a primary sensory tool for receiving information from the environment (Duncan 1978). Many physical injuries are not directly a result of boredom like the examples above, but are a result of the same barren environment that causes the boredom. For instance, wounds on feet and back in pigs are a result of the bare, hard floors (Troxler 1980; Baxter 1981); just as severely damaged claws of hens are caused by the wire floors of battery cages (Tauson 1980). These injuries could be prevented by providing some sort of bedding; this would, at the same time, lead to the alleviation of boredom. The same is true for the tethering of sows; the many traumatic injuries attributed to tethering (Ekesbo 1981a) could be prevented by housing the sows in a free-range pen. The close correlation between understimulation and injury, due to the same practice, indicates the general inadequacy and undesirability of that practice.

GENERAL EVALUATION

Studies described in this chapter about the influence of straw for pigs and deep litter for laying hens confirm the idea that environmental enrichment will be beneficial and adequate as a remedy against some forms of abnormal behaviour.

Is it important to consider boredom seriously as a criterion of welfare, and what its impact is compared to other welfare criteria?

An essential characteristic of boredom in evaluating welfare is that it directly refers to the mental state of the animal and therefore directly implies suffering. Productivity and reproduction are indirect parameters; they are not only animal centered, since the farmer's well-being depends on good productivity as well. Physical injury and disease are animal centered, and it is generally accepted that these are adverse to the animals' mental well-being. If not too severe, and not too prolonged, however, pain and disease might be "bearable." The same may be the case with many forms of stress as a result of overstimulation, since they are temporary and do not fundamentally impair the integrity of the whole animal. But boredom as it is present in today's production system causes the animals to suffer on their most existential level. An animal which cannot express its specific behaviour patterns loses its fundamental selfhood, cannot develop itself in relation to its environment and cannot bear anything, pain in particular. *Deprivation of selfhood is the most fundamental affliction that can be imposed upon an individual, be it pig, chicken or human.*

In nature, animals are never bored. A certain amount of environmental and social stress might be present, but that does not deprive the animal of its capacity to deal with it. If not too severe, it might even enhance its coping abilities. Weather conditions and social interaction are factors that might be desirable in husbandry systems as well. In human society, prisons are confinement systems where material care is sufficient, but the freedom of self-expression is intentionally restricted. This may be a moral choice, but we certainly do not consider a prison a normal environment, and boredom is known to be a chronic problem there.

To suggest that boredom might be fundamentally worse than several forms of pain does not imply, of course, that the infliction of pain should not be avoided where possible. It is not a matter of either one *or* the other. Rather, as has been discussed in this paper, it is very likely that many other welfare characteristics will be improved as well by alleviating boredom. Production, reproduction, and health can be directly improved, because there is either a direct causal relationship between boredom and these characteristics, or there is a positive correlation, as between boredom and physical injury, both being the result of the same causal factor.

The fact that boredom does have quite a wide range of effects on other aspects of the individual animal, shows that it is not just anthropomorphic to state that boredom is fundamentally harmful to the integrity of an animal. Its complete physical health is affected and the deprivation of selfhood is one of the most serious attacks on mental health. This is not an anthropomorphic statement, but a statement about the quality of life, and therefore applying to all living beings.

CONCLUSIONS

1. *An empathetic, caring relationship* between observer and animal is fundamental if we are aiming at knowledge of the subjective experience of the animal under certain conditions. This can be a "personal" relationship between the observer and an individual animal, but it can also take the form of a general empathetic attitude towards a group of animals, or towards lower, less individuated animals.

A detached, dualistic relationship can be regarded as resulting from an interest in knowledge for the sake of manipulation; an attitude of (nonpossessive) love on the other hand has the intention of knowing an object in order to be able to facilitate that the object can truly be or become itself. Therefore, *an empathetic attitude may be more "objective" than a detached one* (see also Section II, *Empathy, Humaneness and Animal Welfare*). Furthermore, the alienation between knower and known is replaced by involvement, and quality becomes more important than quantity because an attitude of care regards an animal as a qualitative being instead of a quantifiable mechanism.

2. Each animal exists on its *own level of beingness*, implying that awareness and emotional experience are fundamental characteristics of life, existing down to the lowest levels. However far removed from human inner experience as the lower levels might be, the concept of beingness implies a respect for the selfhood of each species, and a recognition of the fact that the quality of life matters to each animal.

Many higher vertebrates, such as dogs, dolphins, elephants, primates, etc., show capacities which indicate *self-awareness and a well-developed individual emotional life*. They are intelligent and sensitive and an adequate environment is crucial for the proper expression of their selfhood. We should therefore be prepared to meet animals on their own terms in order to value their innate abilities and potentialities, instead of forcing them to "adapt" to man-made environments and to those conditions that cause them otherwise avoidable stress and distress.

3. Behaviour is the qualitative expression of an animal's selfhood, and is therefore an end in itself, and not a means towards a homeostatic state, or towards successful reproduction. Each animal has basic, genetically inherited, behavioural needs which clearly matter to it, because when it is prevented from performing these behaviours it resorts to abnormal behaviour or becomes apathetic. *An animal can be said to be bored when it has to adapt to its environment in an abnormal way, indicative of understimulation, in order to maintain its sense of selfhood.* Boredom can be regarded as a form of distress, indicating that an animal is stressed, not due to overstimulation, but due to understimulation.

Behavioural criteria of boredom have been delineated in this paper and it was concluded that behaviour represents a higher level of integration than physiology; it concerns the whole, integrated animal, whereas physiology reflects the interaction of the various (unconscious) parts. Physiological processes are directed at the maintenance of a homeostatic state. This state, however, is *not* necessarily equivalent to a state of well-being. Boredom is a form of suffering which primarily is the result of a cognitive process, directly linked to the behavioural possibilities an animal has. Physiological observations are not more objective because they are easier to quantify; in contrast with behaviour they miss the direct link to the subjective experience of an animal, and are therefore, secondary though they might be, useful indicators.

4. Many forms of abnormal behaviour in pigs and chickens are described. Their relatedness to boredom appears from the fact that they usually disappear when some form of environmental enrichment takes place, and when the animals are more able to express different behaviours.

For sows and piglets, the fulfillment of basic needs which prevent the worst forms of boredom seem to be: the ability to *move* unrestrictedly in a certain amount of space; the provision of *straw* and *contact* with other conspecifics.

For chickens, these needs are: some space to *move*, material to perform basic *nest building* behaviour and the opportunity to *search for food* on the floor.

In a housing system where food and drink are provided, the most important remedy against boredom is the provision of explorative possibilities. *Doing something,* whether it be playing, looking for food, or building a nest, constitutes the basis for selfhood. Deprivation of selfhood is the most fundamental affliction for any living being, and is reflected in lower production, lower reproduction, higher disease susceptibility and an increasing amount of physical injury.

Recent research projects indicate that it is possible indeed to create environments for domestic animals which give them much more freedom to express their behavioural needs, within economic limits (Wood-Gush and Stolba 1982; Albright 1982). The argument that if an animal is productive it surely is healthy and adapted, obscures the fact that the use of medical drugs is essential to keep farm animals alive and productive (Fox 1983a). Medical care is very expensive, and the cart is constantly put before the horse in this way. Instead of starting to care for animals when it is almost too late, it seems better to accept care as *the foundation* for our attitude towards them.

In this paper I wanted to indicate and elaborate on the idea that there is an important and direct link between a meta-scientific starting point of empathetic relationship, and practical guidelines for animal husbandry. The willingness to meet animals in a relationship of friendship, thereby discovering their inner world, can result in useful, animal-centered knowledge of their needs and preferences. We might in this way be able to create an environment for the animal which is healthy, both physically and mentally, and which will benefit not only them, but ourselves as well.

REFERENCES

Albright, J.L. 1982. Production changes improve cow veal welfare. *Feedstuffs* April 12:23-33.

American Society of Agricultural Engineers. 1981. Engineering perspectives on farm animal care. Paper no. 81-4580.

Assem, J. van den 1973. Gedrag als aanpassingsfenomeen, een beschouwing over de functie van gedra. In: *Ethologie, de biologie van gedrag*. Pudco, Wageningen. pp. 17-39.

Baldwin, B.A. and Stephens, D.B. 1971. The effects of conditioned behaviour and environmental factors on plasma corticosteroid levels in pigs. *Physiology and Behaviour.* 10:267-74.

Bareham, J.R. 1972. Effects of cages and semi-intensive deep litter pens on the behaviour, adrenal response and production in two strains of laying hens. *Br.Vet.J.* 128:153-63.

Bareham, J.R. 1976. A comparison of the behaviour and production of laying hens in experimental and conventional battery cages. *Applied Animal Ethology* 2:291-303.

Bareham, J.R. and Vestergaard, K. 1981. Welfare and productivity. In: *Research and development in relation to farm animal welfare.* Basel: Birkhäuser Verlag.

Barnett, J.L., Hemsworth, P.H. and Hand, A.M. 1982/83. Effects of chronic stress on some blood parameters in the pig. *Applied Animal Ethology* 9:273-7.

Baxter, S.H. 1981. Welfare and the housing of the sow and suckling pigs. In: Sybesma, W., ed. *The welfare of pigs.* The Hague: Martinus Nijhoff.

Baxter, M.R. 1982/83. Ethology in environmental design for animal production. *Applied Animal Ethology* 9:207-20.

Beilharz, R.G. 1982. Genetic adaptation in relation to animal welfare. *Int.J.Stud.Anim. Prob.* 3(2):117-24.

Beuving, G. 1980. Corticosteroids in laying hens. In: Moss, R., ed. *The laying hen and its environment.* The Hague: Martinus Nijhoff.

Bessei, W. 1980. In: Moss, R., ed. *The laying hen and its environment.* The Hague: Martinus Nijhoff.

Boice, R. 1981. Captivity and feralization. *Psychological Bulletin* 89(3):407-21.

Brantas, G.C. 1975. Welzijn, productie en profijt. *Tijdschr. Diergeneesk.* deel 100(13): 703-8.

Brantas, G.C. 1980. The pre-laying behaviour of laying hens in cages with and without laying nests. In: Moss, R., ed. *The laying hen and its environment.* The Hague: Martinus Nijhoff.

Buchenauer, D. 1981. Parameters for assessing welfare, ethological criteria. In: Sybesma, W., ed. *The welfare of pigs.* The Hague: Martinus Nijhoff.

Buré, R.G. 1981a. Animal well-being and housing systems for piglets. In: Sybesma, W., ed. *The welfare of pigs.* The Hague: Martinus Nijhoff.

Buré, R.G. 1981b. In: Sybesma, W., ed. *The welfare of pigs.* The Hague: Martinus Nijhoff. General discussion, p. 136.

Cassel, E.J. 1982. The nature of suffering and the goals of medicine. *N.Engl.J.Med.* 306:639-45.

Cave, G.P. 1982. Animals, Heidegger and the right to live. *Environmental Ethics*4(3): 249-54.

Craig, J.V. 1982. Behavioral and genetic adaptation of laying hens to high density environments. *Bioscience* 32(1):33-7.

Daelemans, J. 1981. The impact of the farrowing pen on the sow and her piglets. In: Sybesma, W., ed. *The welfare of pigs.* The Hague: Martinus Nijhoff.

Dantzer, R. 1981. In: Sybesma, W., ed. *The welfare of pigs.* The Hague: Martinus Nijhoff. General discussion, p. 133.

Dantzer, R. and Mormède, P. 1979. Le stress en elevage intensif. *Actualités scientifiques et agronomiques* no. 3. Masson, Paris.

Dantzer, R. and Mormède, P. 1981. Can physiological criteria be used to assess welfare in pigs? In: Sybesma, W., ed. *The welfare of pigs.* The Hague: Martinus Nijhoff.

Daschbach, N.J., Schein, M.W. and Haines, D.E. 1982/83. Cage-size effect on locomotor, grooming and agonistic behaviours of the slow loris, *Nycticebus coucang* (primates, Lorisidae). *Applied Animal Ethology* 9:317–30.

Dawkins, M.S. 1980. *Animal suffering: The science of animal welfare.* London, New York: Chapman and Hall.

Debrock, G. 1982. Wisenschaft als Ethik. Manuscript of lecture at Bocholt (Germany).

Duncan, I.J.H. 1973. Can the psychologist measure stress? *The New Scientist* 18 Oct:173–5.

Duncan, I.J.H. 1978. Overall assessment of poultry welfare. In: *Proceedings First Danish Seminar on Poultry Welfare in Egglaying Cages.* pp. 79–87.

Duncan, I.J.H. 1979. Can scientific research help in assessment of animal welfare? In: Proceedings of a symposium held at the University of New England, Armidale, Australia. pp. 169–74.

Duncan, I.J.H. 1981. Animal behaviour and welfare. In: Clark, J.A., ed. *Environmental aspects of housing for animal production.* London: Butterworths.

Ekesbo, I. 1981a. Some aspects of sow health and housing. In: Sybesma, W., ed. *The welfare of pigs.* The Hague: Martinus Nijhoff.

Ekesbo, I. 1981b. In: Sybesma, W., ed. *The welfare of pigs.* The Hague: Martinus Nijhoff. General discussion, p. 233.

Ewbank, R. 1973. Use and abuse of the term "Stress" in husbandry and welfare. *Vet.Rec.* June 30:709–10.

Ewbank, R. 1981. In: Wood-Gush, D.G.M., Dawkins, M., Ewbank, R., eds. *Self-awareness in domesticated animals.* Hertfordshire: UFAW. General discussion, p. 50.

Fauré, J.M. 1980. To adapt the environment to the bird, or the bird to the environment? In: Moss, R., ed. *The laying hen and its environment.* The Hague: Martinus Nijhoff Publishers.

Fölsch, D.W. 1980. Essential behavioural needs. In: Moss, R., ed. *The laying hen and its environment.* The Hague: Martinus Nijhoff.

Fox, M.W. 1971. Psychopathology in man and lower animals. *J.A.V.M.A.* 159(1):66–77.

Fox, M.W. 1974. *Concepts in ethology.* Minneapolis: University of Minnesota Press.

Fox, M.W. 1982. Are most animals "mindless automatons?": A reply to Gordon G. Gallup, Jr. *American J. Primatol.* 3:341–3.

Fox, M.W. 1983a. *Farm animals: husbandry, behavior, and veterinary care: Viewpoints of a critic.* Baltimore: University Park Press.

Fox, M.W. 1983b. Scientific objectivity and the subjective world. In: Rowan, A., ed. *Animal awareness—human perceptions: Implications for animal welfare.* Albany, New York: In press.

Fraser, A.F. 1968. Behaviour disorders in domestic animals. In: Fox, M.W., ed. *Abnormal behaviour in animals.* Philadelphia, London: W.B. Saunders Co.

Fraser, A.F. 1980. Ethology, welfare and preventive medicine for livestock. *Applied Animal Ethology* 6:103–9.

Fraser, D., Ritchie, J.S.D. and Fraser, A.F. 1975. The term stress in a veterinary context. *Br.Vet.J.* 131:653–61.

Freeman, B.M. 1975. Physiological basis of stress. In: *Proceedings of the Royal Society of Medicine* 68:427–9.

Freeman, B.M. 1976. Stress and domestic fowl. A physiological reappraisal. *World Poultry Science Journal* 32(3):249–57.

Freeman, B.M. 1978. Stress in caged layers. In: *The First Danish Seminar on Poultry Welfare in Egglaying Cages.* pp. 57-61.
Friend, T.H. 1980. Stress: What is it, and how can it be quantified? *Int.J.Stud.Anim. Prob.* 1(6):366-74.
Gilson, E. 1976. Descartes: Discours de la méthode; texte et commentaire. 5me edition. *Librairie Philosophique. J. Vrin.* Paris.
Griffin, D.R. 1977. Whitehead's philosophy and some general notions of physics and biology. In: Cobb, J.B. and Griffin, D.R., eds., *Mind in nature.* Washington, D.C.: University Press of America.
Griffin, D.R. 1981a. *The question of animal awareness.* 2nd ed. New York: Rockefeller University Press.
Griffin, D.R. 1981b. The problem of distinguishing awareness from responsiveness. In: Wood-Gush, D.G.M., Dawkins, M. and Ewbank, R., eds. *Self-awareness in domesticated animals.* Hertfordshire: UFAW.
Hammer, W., 1980. Einfluss von Tierbetreuer und Haltungsverfahren auf die Gewichtsentwicklung von Ferkeln. In: *KTBL-Schrift 264. Aktuelle Arbeiten zur artgemässen Tierhaltung.* Darmstadt-Kranichstein.
Hughes, B.O. 1978. Behaviour in different environments and its implications for welfare. In: *The First Danish Seminar on Poultry Welfare in Egglaying Cages.* pp. 21-27.
Hughes, B.O. 1980. The assessment of behavioural needs. In: Sybesma, V., ed. *The laying hen and its environment.* The Hague: Martinus Nijhoff.
Humphrey, N. 1981. In: Wood-Gush, D.G.M., Dawkins, M. and Ewbank, R., eds. *Self-awareness in domesticated animals.* Hertfordshire: UFAW. General discussion, pp. 10, 50.
Ingram, D.L. 1981. In: Sybesma, W., ed. *The welfare of pigs.* The Hague: Martinus Nijhoff.
Kiley-Worthington, M. 1981. In: Wood-Gush, D.G.M., Dawkins, M., Ewbank, R., eds. *Self-awareness in domesticated animals.* Hertfordshire: UFAW. General discussion, p. 50.
Koomans, P. 1981. Open front piggeries with and without straw. In: Sybesma, W., eds. *The welfare of pigs.* The Hague: Martinus Nijhoff.
Lean, I.J. 1978. The pig industry. In: *The welfare of food-animals.* Hertfordshire: UFAW.
Lorz, A. 1979. Tierschutzgesetz. Kommentar. Verl. C.H. Beck, München.
Manning. A. 1972. *An introduction to animal behaviour.* 2nd. ed. London: Edward Arnold Ltd.
Markowitz, H. 1982. *Behavioural enrichment in the zoo.* New York, London: Van Nostrand Reinhold Co.
McBride, G. 1979. Adaptation and welfare at the man-animal interface. Proceedings of a symposium held at the University of New England, Armidale NSW Australia pp. 195-9.
Meijer-Holzapfel, M. 1968. Abnormal behaviour in zoo-animals. In: Fox, M.W., ed. *Abnormal behaviour in animals.* Philadelphia, London: W.B. Saunders Co.
Metz, J.H.M. and Oosterlee, C.C. 1980. Immunologische und ethologische Kriterien für artgemässe Haltung von Sauen und Ferkeln. In: *KTBL-schrift 264.* Aktuelle Arbeiten zure artegemässen Tierhaltung, Darmstadt-Kranichstein.
Moss, B.W. 1981a. The development of a blood profile for stress assessment. In: Sybesma, W., ed. *The welfare of pigs.* The Hague: Martinus Nijhoff.
Moss, B.W. 1981b. In: Sybesma, W., ed. *The welfare of pigs.* The Hague: Martinus Nijhoff. General discussion, p. 137.
Murphy, L.B. 1978. A review of animal welfare and intensive animal production. *Report of the Poultry Section,* Queensland Department of Primary Industries, Australia.

Perry, G. 1973. Can the physiologist measure stress? *The New Scientist* 60:175-7.
Putten, G. van. 1981. Het meten van welzijn bij landbouwhuisdieren *Tijdschr. Diergeneesk* 106(3):106-18.
Putten, G. van. 1982a. De zeugenhouderij. In: *Studiecommisie intensieve veehouderij; fokzeugen, achtste rapport, hoofdstuk* 2. Ned.Ver.tot Besch.v.Dieren, Den Haag.
Putten, G. van. 1982b. Welzijnsaspecten. In: *Studiecommissie intensieve veehouderij: fokzeugen, achtse rapport, hoofstuk* 4. De Haag: Ned. Ver. tot Besch. v. Dieren.
Putten, G. van, and Dammers, J. 1976. A comparative study of the well-being of piglets reared conventionally and in cages. *Applied Animal Ethology* 2:339-56.
Raymond, W.F. 1980. In: Moss, R., ed. *The laying hen and its environment.* The Hague: Martinus Nijhoff. Summary, p. 323.
Sainsbury, M.A. 1978. The poultry industry. In: *The welfare of food animals.* Proceedings of a symposium by UFAW, Hertfordshire, pp. 51-59.
Sambraus, H.H. 1981. Beurteilung von Verhaltens-anomalien aus ethologisher Sicht. 2 GFT-*Seminar für angewandte Nutztierethologie Bayerische Landesanstalt für Tierzucht.* Grub: 1-9.
Sambraus, H.H. 1982. Ethologische Grundlage einer Tiergerechten Nutztierhaltung. In: *Ethologische Aussagen zure artgerechten Nutzierhaltung.* Birkhauser Verlag, Basel. pp. 22-41.
Seligman, M.E.P. 1975. *Helplessness.* San Francisco: W.H. Freeman and Co.
Siegel, H.S. 1980. Physiological stress in birds. *Bioscience* 30:529-34.
Stolba, A. and Wood-Gush, D.G.M. 1980. Arousal and exploration in growing pigs in different evironments. *Applied Animal Ethology* 6(4):382-3.
Stolba, A. 1982. Wild pigs point the way. *Animal Welfare Institute Quarterly.* 31(1):7.
Tauson, R. 1980. Cages: how could they be improved? In: Moss, R., ed. *The laying hen and its environment.* The Hague: Martinus Nijhoff.
Tranøy, K.E. 1977. Three thoughts about objectivity as a methodological norm. In: *Danish Yearbook of Philosophy,* Vol.14. Munksgaard, Copenhagen.
Troxler, J. 1980. Beurteilung zweier Haltungssysteme für Absatzferkel. In: *KTBL-schrift 264, Aktuelle Arbeiten zur artgemässen Tierhaltung,* Darmstadt-Kranichstein.
Truyen, W.T. 1981. In: Sybesma, W., ed. *The Welfare of Pigs.* The Hague: Martinus Nijhoff. General discussion, pp. 232-3.
Verhoog, H. 1983. De relatie tussen biologie en menswetenschappen. Manuscript.
Vestergaard, K. 1981. Influence of fixation on the behaviour of sows. In: Sybesma, W., ed. *The welfare of pigs.* The Hague: Martinus Nijhoff.
Wemelsfelder, F. 1982. Gedrag als mogelijke indicator voor pijn bij biggen. Verslag van onderzoeksstage 109, IVO-Zeist. Niet voor publicatie.
Wiepkema, P.R. 1980. Ein biologische modell von Verhaltenssystemen. In: *KTBL-schrift 264,* Aktuelle Arbeiten zur artgemässen Tierhaltung, Darmstadt-Kranichstein.
Wiepkema, P.R. 1982. On the identity and significance of disturbed behaviour in verterbrates. In: Bessei, W., ed. *Disturbed behaviour in farm animals.* Hohenheimer Arbeiten, Heft 121: Eugen Ulmer Verlag, Stuttgart.
Wood-Gush, D.G.M. 1973. Animal welfare in modern agriculture, *Br.Vet.J.* 129:164-74.
Wood-Gush, D.G.M. 1981. In: Wood-Gush, D.G.M., Dawkins, M., Ewbank, R. eds. *Self-awareness in domesticated animals.* Hertfordshire: UFAW. General discussion.
Wood-Gush, D.G.M. and Stolba, A. 1982. Behaviour of pigs and the design of a new housing system. *Applied Animal Ethology* 8(6):583-4.
Zuriff, G. 1982. A dog remembers. *The Sciences.* Dec.:10-11. New York: The New York Academy of Sciences.

EVILS OF MODERN STABLES*

James Irvine Lupton
(1884)

INTRODUCTION

Portions of veterinarian James Irvine Lupton's book on horse management that deal with the problems of confinement husbandry practices have been selected as a significant historical record of humane concerns that were documented one hundred years ago. While the author's descriptive prose may lack scientific "objectivity," it does express a common sense morality and the subjective and intuitive observations and conclusions of an experienced veterinarian who clearly respects and understands the horse. His words bespeak of a bygone era where the care or husbandry of animals was both an art and a science, a discipline based upon empathy, compassion and factual knowledge. How far indeed have we progressed, ethically and technologically, in improving the husbandry of domesticated animals, such as the horse, since 1884? While conditions may be more sanitary and diseases better understood, prevented, and treated, it is a fact that stabled horses in 1984 are too often kept under comparable conditions of extreme deprivation and show the same behavioral pathologies that Lupton so clearly describes.

M.W. Fox
Editor

**From Mayhew's Illustrated Horse Management (1884), revised and improved by James Irvine Lupton, M.R.C.V.S., author of several works on veterinary science and art. London: Wm. H. Allen & Co., 13, Waterloo Place Pall Mall, S.W.*

THE EVILS WHICH ARE OCCASIONED BY MODERN STABLES

It does not require any vast expenditure of thought to discover that life is action; "to be," is synonymous with "to do": therefore, it is a sheer necessity of existence that an animated being must be doing something. Such is the primary consequence of existence. Thus, to breathe and to move imply one act; since, if the lungs cease to dilate, respiration immediately terminates, and, with it, animation comes to an end. Yet, it remained for mortal perversity to rebuke the first principle of established philosophy, when stables were built, in which a breathing animal was to be treated as it were an inanimate chattel.

Nature, like a kind mother, is to this day endeavouring to teach her wayward children a plain truth, which they may hourly behold enforced by visible examples. The wilful brood appears to be in no hurry to learn. Man still treats the horse as though he honoured the quadruped by enslaving it; and ennobled a life, by conferring upon the animal the title of his servant. He acts as though, by such conduct, sufficient reason were exhibited why he should oblige the creature to resign its instincts and relinquish its desires.

The equine race, when in a wild state, are gregarious, or congregate in herds. Man captures such a quadruped and places it in a stable, built to enforce the extreme of solitary confinement. The plain is the natural abode of the herd; on their speed depend both their pleasure and their safety. Man ties the domesticated horse to a manger, and pays a groom to enforce absolute stagnation upon innate activity. The "panting steed" is the most timid of living beings. Man insists the charger is possessed of extraordinary courage; he declares it delights in the tumult of battle; and he esteems it a glorious achievement to brutally coerce the timorous sensibility. The mild-eyed horse is, perhaps, the most simple of all the breathing beauties which adorn a wondrous world. Man declares all of the gentle breed have dangerous propensities, and are most inherently vicious.

Before subjugation, the creature fed off the surface of the earth. Man builds a house specially designed for the captive, in which the corn is placed on a level with the chest, and the hay is stationed as high up as the head. The animal is gifted with affections; it longs to gratify their promptings; it yearns for something upon which its abundant love may gush forth,—a fellow-prisoner—a goat—a dog—a cat—a fowl;—no matter what,—so it be some living object, on which may be lavished that excess of tenderness which, confined to its own breast, renders being miserable. Man esteems it his primary duty to clear the stable of all possible companionship; but the creature which would rejoice, were it only permitted to worship its enslaver, he rarely approaches without a loud voice, a harsh word, or a harsher blow, announcing his presence to the captive.

The inhabitant of such a prison, a domesticated horse miserably drags through a shortened life, under human *protection*. The nearest approach it can make to freedom is its period of labour. It always rejoices to quit its confinement; but, enfeebled by imprisonment, and subservient to man's exactions, it ever gladly returns to the place of its sorrow. In proportion as its limbs are finely made, and its actions are graceful, is it prized. It is never esteemed for its instincts, or credited with intelligence. It lives in so limited a space, that, in comparison with the dimensions of its abode, a man in a sentry-box dwells in a mansion; or a lion in a cage roams over a domain. A reasonable and an intelligent being commands his horse should be fastened to such a spot, and supposes that a living organism is to endure the confinement, which does not permit the body to turn round; that animated functions are to exist where most ordinary exercises are rendered impossible: nevertheless, he anticipates the creature will appear bounding with health, in answer to his requirements.

To be sure the prisoner, although its head be fastened (a restraint not imposed upon the most savage of carnivorous beasts), is permitted now to bear upon one leg, and then to change it for the other. It may perhaps lie down or stand up, without provoking chastisement. Neither head nor tail is forbidden a *proper* degree of motion. But at this point all indulgence is exhausted. It is tied to a rope two yards in length; but it may not go even to the extent of its tether; neither may it move close up to the manger; both acts are equally unpardonable: a properly behaved animal should stand quietly in the centre of its compartment, and always remain there when not lying down.

It is beaten, if its head be raised just to peep over the paling, to exchange a rub of the nose and to give, as well as accept, a warm stream of fragrant breath to and from its nearest fellow-misery. It must taste the full flavour of its captivity: no trivial act may distract attention from the horror of its position. It must lie down where it stands; and stand where it laid down. It must not display the grace and ease of motion with which it has been endowed; nor must it indulge the kindly feelings Providence has gifted it with. If the owner of the horse does not recognize the exquisite adaptation of sight, so as to infract the minutest particle, and to view the most distant object, the sensibility of hearing to which movements are audible, when to the duller perceptions of man no sound vibrates on the air; the keenness of scent, which can appreciate qualitites in substances which to human sense are devoid of odour; the fleetness of motion which was permitted as a protection, the ease of which the most perfect machinery has failed to rival;—how can he expect his servant to inquire whether such attributes were given by Nature, only to be fastened by the head or to be confined within a space in which absolute stagnation must ultimately induce bodily incapacity.

Such a true "Vis inertiae" can alone be varied by the hours of labour and the periods of feeding. All pastime is unlawful; the most innocent amusement must be practised silently and in secret. Certain animals, however, try to get through the long hours of enforced idleness by quietly nibbling at the topmost rail of the manger. Large portions of tough wood are often removed after this fashion; and, to him who can rightly interpret signs, a thick post bitten away, fibre by fibre, will present melancholy evidence of that longing for employment, which could induce so great a waste of perseverance; for animals are naturally great economists of labour.

Other prisoners will endeavour to cheat the time by licking their mangers, apparently in the hope that some stray grain of corn may have escaped previous attention. The soft tongue of the horse, passed over the hardened surface of the wood, occasions no noise. Often a few grains will have lodged in the corners; then the effort to displace these affords a long game. Others, from want of something to do, or from finding impure air and inactivity do not, in accordance with the general doctrine, promote equine digestion, learn "to crib;" a few, from the operation of the like causes, become perfect as "wind suckers." All "speed the weary hours" as they best can; and many heads are turned around to discover if it be feeding-time again; not that they are hungry, but eating is an occupation, and they sadly wish for some employment.

Certain quadrupeds, under these circumstances, adopt a habit, which is the more remarkable, because hours of tedium have generated the like indulgence in human beings. Mortals, when compelled to remain stationary, and forced to preserve silence, often strive to kill time by rocking to and fro, or by "see-sawing" their bodies. Such a pitiable excuse for amusement is very common among the little people whose undeveloped limbs are perched on high forms, and in whose hands are fixed very uninteresting primers, from which the infant mind wanders into vacuity during the hours of imprisonment which occur in those pleasing places termed "Preparatory Schools." The horse, also, when forbidden the pleasures in which Nature formed it to delight, will move its head methodically from one side of its stall to the other, and will continue thus engaged for hours together.

So exciting a pastime, most sane people might deem to be harmless enough; but by the arbitrary notions of rectitude entertained within the stable such custom is punished as a vice. A horse which "see-saws" is said to weave, and weaving is, by grooms, esteemed highly culpable, and is usually corrected with the lash.

Can human perversity conceive a life without a pastime, and vexatiously impose this terrible fate upon the creature whose existence is devoted to man's service? When in the field, the horse is never idle. The only amusement of the simple animal lies in its perpetual occupation. What a despairing sorrow must therefore afflict such an existence, when dragging through its time under the fostering care of the enslaver. Yet how proudly do some intellectual beings boast of their stables and of the ceaseless attention lavished on their studs. What is it this assiduity realizes to the creature on which it is expended? Stagnation to the active, and solitude to the gregarious. Movement draws down punishment, as it were a fault. Any attempt to while away the tedious hours is esteemed "a vice"; sensation must be checked, and feeling, man insists shall be suppressed. But who, among the millions of intellectual masters, sufficiently understands the quadruped, over which they all usurp authority, to regard the huge bulk of that endurance, as the embodiment of the acutest form of every possible earthly misery?

Perpetual inaction also occasions waste of food: the horse, wanting exercise, stares at his provender, but has no appetite; the hay piled up before it is nothing more than matter out of place.

Desire is needed to give value to such abundance; and a non-reasoning being cannot be expected to prize that which it does not require. It cannot eat; but it lacks amusement. The hay is before it. In sheer idleness, a few stalks are pulled from the rack. Of these, one may be leisurely masticated; but the remainder, after having been twisted about the lips, are allowed to fall upon the litter. The sport is followed up until the rack is emptied; and the creature is a little happier, under a conviction that it has escaped from absolute stagnation.

The sin, if there be any, certainly must remain with the man who piled up the provender before the animal which was without an appetite.

Simple natures, when entirely disengaged, generally make their own employment, and that employment, being intended for a passing amusement, commonly consists of what thrifty people designate "mischief." The knowledge, that displeasure will follow upon discovery, may spice the proceeding which otherwise might want interest. At all events, so it is with children; and it may be thus with animals. When a heaped manger is before a satiated quadruped, the impossibility of feeding makes the creature meditate upon the uses to which the grain can possibly be applied. None can be discovered. The head of the captive is tied, and the manger is fixed. At length, in carelessness of spirit, a mouthful is taken from the heap. The portion cannot be swallowed, so the lips are moved, and, as they part, the corn falls over them upon the ground. This may not be a very exciting recreation; but the prisoner is restless with repletion. It cannot sleep; and the grain passing over the lips, in which equine feeling concentrates, produces a slight and a novel sensation.

Can any man seriously pronounce that an animal, standing in enforced solitude and compulsory idleness, is to blame for such conduct? Boys, during their school days, when wanting appetite, or having unnecessary food before them, will not they, in satiety, play with needless abundance? Are men to demand that prudence from an animal, which we should certainly not anticipate in the young of our own species? Yet the child enjoys a certain amount of confidence; and its misdoing is, therefore, aggravated by a certain abuse of trust. The horse is confined between boards, and enjoys not the smallest personal liberty. The severity of captivity argues, that no reliance reposes upon the captive's discretion. All responsibility is lost when all freedom of action is denied. Yet the poor prisoner is cruelly beaten for playing with food, although the true fault rested upon him who was too idle to give the exercise which would have generated appetite; and was too lazy to proportion the animal's sustenance to the requirments of its situation.

Another so-named "vice" of the horse is frequently the occasion of more serious results than any of the before-mentioned accidents. No person has hitherto explained why the skin should be more irritable by night than during the daytime. Such, however, is the case with horses, as it is with men. A quadruped, in the morning, is often found disfigured by the hair being removed from comparatively large surfaces. Itchiness has provoked the animal to rub itself against any prominence, or to scratch its body with the toe of its iron shoe; this indulgence has caused the blemish.

Itching and scratching are numbered among the worst "vices" of the stable. Such faults, however, are only discovered in their effects; the groom never estimates, when flogging an animal for this wickedness, how far the abhorred sin may have been produced by stimulating diet, by want of exercise, and by impure atmosphere. No! he clothes up the body of the animal; shuts every window; stops every cranny; and locks the stable door for the night. The last meal being consumed, and the quadrupeds not being inclined for sleep, they one and all begin to itch. Legs are nibbled; necks are rubbed; and tails are lashed. At length one is sensible of an irritation behind the ear. The head is turned toward the side; the body is curved to the full extent; and the hind leg brought forward. Then, the groom not being present, the toe of the hind shoe can touch the part, and the horse luxuriates in a hearty titillation.

When the head was turned toward the quarters, however, the collar-rope, being attached to the halter, was also stretched in that direction. The hind foot having performed its office, a desire is felt to return to the natural position. The attempt is made; but this is found to be impracticable. The creature strains against the opposing force, but its struggles only render its comfortless attitude the more fixed. The truth is, that while devoted to the act which allays cuticular irritability, the pastern has slipped over the collar-rope. Such a mishap not only fixes the leg, but fastens the head. With the neck bent and one leg disabled, the animal cannot exert half its power; neither can simplicity comprehend the source of its unnatural constraint. Long continuance of the position becomes painful; alarm seizes upon timidity; the struggles grow desperate; and the poor quadruped, at length, is cast with terrible violence upon the straw which had been shaken down for its repose.

The strongest testimony, however, against stables, as such buildings are at present erected, is perhaps borne by the animals which inhabit those places. The horse is a delicate test, which man would do well to attentively observe when he is desirous of ascertaining the healthfulness of any locality. Naturally it is all animation and gaiety of spirit. But, however much these qualities may be esteemed, such equine recommendations will soon fade before the joint influence of impure air and close confinement, although you may groom and feed at discretion. The natural period of life is diminished one half, while much more than half of the remaining years is rendered useless by age, prematurely brought on by inappropriate treatment.

STEREOTYPE BEHAVIOUR IN SOWS AND GILTS HOUSED IN STALLS, TETHERS, AND GROUPS

Judith K. Blackshaw* and J.F. McVeigh**

**Department of Animal Production*
University of Queensland,
St. Lucia, Queensland, 4067
(Australia)

***Piggery Manager, Veterinary Science Farm*
University of Queensland
Moggill Road
Pinjarra Hills, Queensland, 4069
(Australia)

ABSTRACT

Observations of sows and gilts in tethers, stalls, and groups showed two distinct types of behaviour: pre-feed behaviour when pigs were anticipating food, and after-feed behaviour. Sows and gilts tethered for the first time do not show pre-feed excitement, but this develops in 42 days which suggests that pre-feed behaviour is not stereotype, as suggested by the literature, but is a conditioned reflex.

The question of the importance of after-feeding behaviours which are often called stereotypies is examined. The total time occupied by these behaviours over 24 hours by tethered sows is 14.5 to 29.0%, by tethered gilts 1.4 to 5.6%, by stalled sows 10 to 14%, and 4.2 to 6.3% in stalled gilts.

Grouped animals do not show the same behaviours as the stalled and tethered ones.

Several examples of true stereotypies are described, but not all tethered or stalled pigs exhibit chronic bar biting. Changes in the environment of two of these sows did not alter the fixed stereotype behaviour. Each individual seems to have an optimum level of environmental stimulation which may account for the great differences in individual behaviours.

INTRODUCTION

Those movements which are combined into rhythmic or complex sequences of obscure purpose are described as stereotypies. Hediger (1955) described stereotypies in caged zoo animals which included weaving to and fro, pacing up and down, and circling.

Removal of the animal from the cage may cause the stereotypy to cease, but this is not always so (Meyer-Holzapfel 1968). Novel objects may initially reduce the performance of stereotypies in horses but this lasts only as long as the object remains novel. In cases where animals have been performing the stereotypies for some time the introduction of a novel object may actually increase the frequency of the stereotypy (Kiley-Worthington 1983).

Some stereotypies may function as an adaptive mechanism and be regarded as the attempt of a normal individual to cope with an abnormal environment (Ridley and Baker 1982). This abnormal environment may result from conflict or frustration situations, low sensory input (boredom state) or very high sensory input (e.g. novel objects).

All these types of situations may contribute at some time to stereotypies reported in farm animals, such as bar-biting in tether stalled pigs (Fraser 1975) and weaving, wind-sucking, and crib-biting in horses (Kiley-Worthington 1983).

Some stereotypies in pigs and horses are performed when food is anticipated (Fraser 1975; Kiley-Worthington 1983). It has been suggested also that rapidly consumed food and the lack of even, low-quality, high fibre food to eat at leisure is a major cause of stereotypies in herbivores (Kiley-Worthington 1983).

Dantzer and Mormède (1981) suggested that pituitary-adrenal activity is a good indicator of emotional arousal. They looked at a chain-pulling stereotypy performed by food deprived pigs who were then submitted to an intermittent food delivery schedule (Dantzer et al. 1980; Dantzer and Mormède 1983). This chain-pulling activity was accompanied by decreased pituitary-adrenal activity which indicates a decrease in tension or anxiety. Their data suggests that stereotypies enable the animals to decrease excessive arousal, rather than provide an extra source of stimulation.

Horse stereotypies show many characteristics of learned behaviour (Kiley-Worthington 1983) which may be evoked by some mild stimulus (head tossing as a result of nasal irritation initially) or learning by imitation, as in some cases of crib-biting.

There is no published evidence for this in pigs but this study suggests there is an element of learning involved in the development of stereotypies. It also examines the behaviour performed by tethered, stalled, and groups of pigs before feeding and after feeding, and comments on the effect of changing the environment on several complex sequences of stereotypic behaviour in sows. Comment is also made on the notable absence of chronic bar-biting in this herd.

MATERIALS AND METHODS

The study was carried out in a 55-sow, specific pathogen-free herd at the Veterinary Science Farm Piggery, University of Queensland (Australia), during 1982-83. The behaviour of the animals (Large White x Landrace) in three husbandry systems for sows and gilts was examined.

(i) Stall system providing 1.04 m^2/pig;

(ii) Neck tether system providing 1.04 m^2/pig; but the 65 cm chain allows each pig to use 3.0 m^2 of space effectively;

(iii) Group system of six pigs in a pen (6.24 m^2).

Flooring was concrete in the stalls, each pig being provided with a concrete trough, concrete floor and slats with a metal trough in the tethers, and concrete floor and slats in the group pens with floor feeding.

Food was provided twice/day at 0800 to 0830 and 1300 to 1350 in the form of pellets.

OBSERVATIONS—EXPERIMENT 1

Two types of observations were made in each husbandry system:

(i) Detailed observations each week on 36 tethered sows, 8 tethered gilts, 9 sows in stalls, 10 gilts in stalls, two groups of 6 gilts, and five groups of 6 sows each, penned.

These observations were made from the time of confirmation of pregnancy when the pigs were put in the husbandry system until farrowing. Detailed observations were made on day 1 and covered the two feeding periods. Subsequent observations were done each week and covered only one feeding period. Behaviour was recorded from the time the pigs anticipated their food (5 to 15 minutes), during the feeding period and until the pigs lay down.

(ii) Surveys of all the pigs in stalls, tethers, and pens with time sampling during both the day and night.

EXPERIMENT 2

Another section of the experiment was to determine how stereotypies develop. The two groups of penned gilts (6 in each group) from the previous experiment were used after farrowing as parity 1 sows and placed in tethers when pregnancy was confirmed. They were observed each week before, during and after a feed period to determine when or if, stereotypies developed.

RESULTS

EXPERIMENT 1

There were two distinct types of behaviour in stalled, tethered, and penned pigs:
(i) Before-feed behaviour, and
(ii) After-feed behaviour.

PENNED SOWS AND GILTS

The grouped sows (five groups of 6 sows) were only kept together for one day over two feeding periods, as the agonistic behaviour (conflict behaviour involving threats, bites, fights) prevented any other behaviour patterns from emerging.

The grouped gilts (two groups of 6 gilts) showed some pre-feed excitement which consisted of crowding and pushing to the fence as the food trolley came past. There was no pawing or head waving nor was there opportunity for any bar-biting. Agonistic activity which occurred over the first 16-minute feed period averaged 4 agonistic incidents/minute. This decreased over the next three months to average 1.8/minute.

Pigs showed no true stereotypies after feeding—the first gilt lay down within 17-34 minutes after the beginning of feeding and all gilts were consistently lying by 76 minutes after feeding. There were examples of gilts who sat and chewed for up to 20 minutes in the after-feed period, but this ceased when they lay down.

STALLS AND TETHERS

Pre-feed behaviour

Pre-feed excitement was shown in stalled sows and gilts, and in tethered sows and gilts when food was anticipated. These behaviours are similar to those described by Fraser (1975), and are listed in Table 1a. Day 1 is the day that the pig is put in the husbandry system and the frequency of the behaviour is noted over the first feeding period. The tethered and stalled sows showed more pre-feed behaviour sequences than the tethered and stalled gilts. Agonistic displays were not evident in tethered gilts, nor in stalled sows or gilts. The agonistic activities in the tethered sows dropped from 47% of all sows over the first two weeks to one example over the three-month period.

Table 1a. Pre-feed behaviours (5 to 12 minutes before feeding) and the frequency they occurred on the first day that sows and gilts are stalled or tethered.

Tether				Stalls			
Sows (36)		Gilts (8)		Sows (9)		Gilts (10)	
Day 1							
Agonistic displays	17*	Stand for feed	5	Yell	7	Stand for feed	6
Yell	26	Lie until feed comes	4	Paw	3	Paw	1
Paw	23	Pull at tether	1	Nosing bars	2	Stand and chew	1
Nosing bars	10			Froth and chew bar	4	Chew bar	1
Froth and chew bar	12			Stand and chew	1	Poke nose in and out front bar	1
Stand and chew	1			Wave head	7		
Stand	6			Poke nose in and out front bar	6		
Wave head	18						

*frequency of behaviour
A pig may show more than one behaviour.

It can be seen (Table 1b) that some of the tethered gilts learned to chew the bar, wave their heads, paw and yell during the succeeding three-month observation period. However, there were 5 gilts who did not show these behaviours and stood up when food was anticipated.

Bar-biting was observed in 17 tethered sows consistently but was interspersed with pawing, yelling and head waving. Some stalled sows

Table 1b. Pre-feed behaviours observed in tethered and stalled sows and gilts over a three-month period.

Tether		Stalls	
Sows (36)	Gilts (8)	Sows (9)	Gilts (10)
Agonistic Displays			
Yell	Stand for feed	Yell	Stand for feed
Paw	Yell	Paw	Paw
Nose bars	Paw	Nose bars	Stand and chew
Froth and chew bar	Nose bar	Froth and chew bar	Chew bar
Stand and chew	Chew bar	Poke nose in and out of front bar	Poke nose in and out of front bar
Wave head	Wave head		

and gilts also bit the bar, but again it was interspersed with other activities.

These behaviours occupied a very small time period over 24 hours. It was 1.7 to 2.0% of the time in stalled and tethered sows, 0 to 0.4% in tethered gilts and 0 to 0.2% in stalled gilts.

Fraser (1975) refers to head waving as a stereotype but it is evident that none of these behaviours are stereotypies when the definition is considered. They are sequences which occur, and indeed might be expected, in animals who are waiting for their hunger to be satisfied.

AFTER-FEED BEHAVIOUR

This is one of the periods when stereotypies are reported to occur in pigs. The behaviours for stalled sows and gilts and tethered sows and gilts until they rest are shown in Table 2. These behaviours occupy between 14.5 to 29.0% of a 24-hour period in tethered sows, 10.0 to 14.0% in stalled sows, 1.4 to 5.6% in tethered gilts and 4.2 to 6.3% in stalled gilts.

There were no examples of chronic bar-biting or the pre-feed behaviours of yell, paw, wave head, but there were several examples of true stereotypies which were performed continuously by individual

Table 2. After-feed behaviours observed in tethered and stalled sows and gilts before rest.

Tether		Stalls	
Sows (36)	Gilts (8)	Sows (9)	Gilts (10)
Lie	Lie	Lie	Lie
Lie and chew	Lie and chew	Lie and chew	Lie and chew
Lick trough	Lick trough	Stand and chew	Stand and chew
Stand and chew	Stand and chew	Lick trough	Sit and chew
Chew trough	Rub nose on floor	Rub nose on trough	Sit
Play with chain		Rub nose on floor	Lick trough
Rub nose on floor			
Rub nose on trough			

pigs until they lay down. These were observed for three months:

(i) A tethered sow who continually pressed the water nozzle and squirted water over the floor in random bursts (45 seconds to 140 seconds with 3- to 5- second stops in between).

(ii) A tethered sow who sat poking her tongue in and out.

(iii) A tethered sow who pushed the water nozzle and licked the water in sequences of 27–30 seconds of continuous pressing, then a rest period of 2 seconds. This was repeated for an average of 165 minutes until the pig lay down.

(iv) A stalled sow who rubbed her nose in an upward direction on the two front bars of her stall in a random pattern which also had a random time component.

Kiley-Worthington (1983) points out that in horses there appears to be an optimum level of environmental stimulation for each individual. This seems to be similar to pigs and may account for the great differences in individual behaviours.

An interesting observation was that when the tethered pig who continually squirted water had farrowed and was placed in stalls she continued this stereotypy. Also the bar rubbing stereotypy described in the stalled sow continued when she was tethered. This indicated that a fixed stereotypy is difficult to stop even by a change of environment.

The frequencies of the other after-feed behaviours are given in the survey results for tethered pigs (Table 3) and stalled pigs (Table 4) which were done in the daytime. A survey of tethered and stalled pigs over 15 hours (1500 - 0645) is shown in Tables 5a and 5b.

One hour after feeding, stand and chew, followed by stand and lick trough, were the most common behaviours. Stand and chew was the most common behaviour for two to three hours following feeding, after which most pigs were resting.

Table 3. Behaviour of 30 tethered pigs on three different days (number indicates the number of pigs performing the behaviour).

	Day 1		Day 2	Day 3	
Behaviour	1 hr before feed (0800)	5–15 min before feed (0845)	3 hr 40 min after feed (1240)	1 hr after feed (1500)	3hr after feed (1700)
Lie only	8	0	8	4	7
Lie and chew	2	0	6	3	4
Stand only	3	6	3	0	0
Stand and chew	8	5	3	9	7
Stand and lick trough	3	2	3	9	4
Sit only	2	1	2	2	0
Sit and chew	0	0	3	2	6
Stand and poke tongue in and out	1	1	1	1	1
Stand with nose pressed on bar	1		0	0	0
Chew bar	1		0	0	0
Stand and head wave	1	2	0	0	0
Stand, wave and paw	0	6	0	0	0
Stand, wave, chew bar	0	3	0	0	0
Stand and paw	0	4	0	0	0
Play with chain	0	0	0	0	1

Table 4. The behaviour of 18 stalled pigs on day 1, and 15 stalled pigs on day 2 (number indicates the number of pigs performing the behaviour).

	Day 1 (18 pigs)			Day 2 (15 pigs)		
Behaviour	5-15 min before feed (0845)	3 hr after feed (1200)	4 hr after feed (1300)	1 hr after feed (1500)	2 hr after feed (1600)	3 hr after feed (1700)
Lie only	0	13	9	1	1	14
Lie and chew	0	0	0	0	0	0
Stand only	5	0	0	2	0	1
Stand and chew	0	5	6	9	11	0
Stand and lick trough	0	0	0	3	2	0
Sit only	0	0	2	0	0	0
Sit and chew	0	0	0	0	0	0
Stand and poke tongue	0	0	0	0	0	0
Nose pressed on bar	0	0	1	0	0	0
Chew bar	4	0	0	0	1	0
Stand head wave	9	0	0	0	0	0
Stand and paw	0	0	0	0	0	0

Table 5a. Behaviours observed in 35 tethered pigs from 1500-0645 hours (15 hr 45 min); fed at 1430 and all pigs lie from 1830 to 0640.

Behaviour	1500	1530	1600	1630	1700	1730	1800	1830	0645*
Lie	3	11	4	16	24	23	33	35	25
Lie and chew	0	0	2	2	2	4	0	0	0
Stand	1	10	19	3	3	4	2	0	7
Stand and chew	1	6	5	0	0	0	0	0	0
Stand and lick trough	29	6	0	10	0	0	0	0	3
Sit	1	1	2	2	5	1	0	0	0
Sit and chew	0	1	3	2	1	3	0	0	0

*The husbandman arrived to feed the pigs.

Table 5b. Behaviours observed in 11 stalled pigs from 1500-0645 hours; fed at 1430, and all pigs rest from 1830 to 0640.

Behaviour	1500	1530	1600	1630	1700	1730	1800	1830	0645*
Lie	5	8	5	8	9	9	5	11	6
Lie and chew	0	0	0	0	0	0	1	0	0
Stand	3	0	0	3	1	0	4	0	3
Stand and chew	1	1	0	0	0	0	0	0	0
Stand and lick trough	2	1	4	0	0	0	0	0	0
Sit	0	1	2	0	0	1	1	0	0
Sit and chew	0	0	0	0	1	1	0	0	2

*The husbandman arrived to feed the pigs.

EXPERIMENT 2

During the first observations after the parity 1 sows settled into their tethers there was not the pre-feed excitement exhibited by the older sows. None of them pawed, waved their heads back and forth, or yelled. These sows had been penned together until parturition and this was their first experience in tethers.

The sows, by 42 days in tethers, were exhibiting some pre-feed excitement by salivating, waving heads, and pushing their snouts through the front bars of the tether-stall.

After-feed behaviour included rubbing snout along the floor under the trough, licking inside the trough and chewing. All sows were lying down by 100 minutes after feeding although there were great individual differences. One sow consistently showed no after-feed behaviour and lay down immediately.

As yet, true stereotype behaviours have not developed in these animals, which suggests that an element of learning is involved in their development.

CONCLUSIONS

Only four examples of true stereotype behaviour appeared which might indicate that these individuals have a different tolerance level to the other animals. Changes in environment did not alter the complex fixed stereotype behaviour in two sows. It is suggested that some stereotype behaviour is conditioned.

The pre-feed excitement is not stereotype behaviour according to the definition, but is a conditioned reflex. Only a few tethered or stalled sows and gilts exhibited chronic bar-biting before or after feeding.

There remains the question of whether the after feeding behaviours observed in most animals are true stereotype behaviours, as described in the literature. It seems unlikely that most of them are harmful to the welfare of the animals in this piggery.

The piggery in this study has several factors which may account for the lack of serious stereotypies:

(i) many students go into the piggery and handle the animals during clinical procedures,

(ii) several ongoing research projects are carried out continuously,

(iii) the husbandman is interested in the pigs' welfare.

If stereotypies are due to boredom and lack of stimulation as has been suggested, the presence of people may prevent this.

EDITORS' ADDENDUM

ANIMAL RIGHTS AND THE NON-THERAPEUTIC USE OF DRUGS

The use of prostaglandins to induce farrowing in pigs (regardless of the stage of farrowing at which different sows might be) is an animal welfare and rights issue. (I am not opposed to valid veterinary use of prostaglandins to help us deal with the reproductive problems of pigs, horses, and other animals that might otherwise jeopardize their health and well-being.) But it is surely ethically questionable to use prostaglandins to make sows *in different stages of labor* give birth at the same time, irregardless of potentially harmful consequences. This is done so that expectant sows will give birth during working hours. While this is consonant with the economic "efficiencies" of the hog factory farm, it certainly is not in accord with the biology and psychology of the sow. Judith Blackshaw has clearly demonstrated, in her research on sows being given prostaglandins near to delivery, that such treatment intensifies instinctual impulses and needs, which can lead to what humanitarians intuit as frustration and distress. The use of antibiotics as feed additives for farm animals and of analgesic drugs to enable injured and lame horses to be raced, are other examples of the unethical and commercial, as distinct from veterinary, use of drugs in animals today, which should be questioned.

REFERENCES

Dantzer, R. and Mormede, P. 1981. Can physiological criteria be used to assess welfare in pigs? *Curr. Topics Vet. Med. Anim. Sci.* 11:53-73.

Dantzer, R. and Mormede, P. 1983. De-arousal properties of stereotyped behaviour: evidence from pituitary-adrenal correlates in pigs. *Appl. Anim. Etho.* 10:233-44.

Dantzer, R., Arnone, M. and Mormède, P. 1980. Effects of frustration on behaviour and plasma corticosteroid levels in pigs. *Physiol. Beha.* 24(1):1-4.

Fraser, D. 1975. The effect of straw on the behaviour of sows in tether stalls. *Anim. Prod.* 21:59-68.

Hediger, H. 1955. *Studies of the psychology and behaviour of captive animals in zoos and circuses.* New York:Criterion Press.

Kiley-Worthington, M. 1983. Stereotypes in horses. *Equine Practice* 5:34-40.

Meyer-Holzapfel, M. 1968. Abnormal behaviour in zoo animals. In: Fox, M.W. ed. *Abnormal behaviour in animals.* Philadelphia:W.B. Saundeson, pp. 476-503.

Ridley, R.M. and Baker, H.F. 1982. Stereotypy in monkeys and humans. *Psychol. Med.* 12:61-72.

Part V
Appendix

AMERICAN ATTITUDES TOWARD AND KNOWLEDGE OF ANIMALS: AN UPDATE*†

Stephen R. Kellert

ABSTRACT

The distribution of a typology of basic attitudes toward animals in the American population is explored through personal interviews with 3,107 randomly selected persons in the 48 contiguous states and Alaska. Data is presented on the prevalence of these attitudes in the overall American population and among major social demographic and animal activity groups. In addition, results are presented on Americans' knowledge of animals as well as their species preferences. Finally, information is presented on perceptions of critical wildlife issues including endangered species, predator control, hunting, trapping, marine mammals and wildlife habitat protection.

INTRODUCTION

During the period 1973-1976, a typology of basic attitudes toward animals was developed and a limited study conducted to examine the distribution of these viewpoints throughout the American public (Kellert 1978). In 1977, the U.S. Fish and Wildlife Service of the Department of the Interior granted funds to explore more carefully the presence and strength of these perceptions among diverse social demographic and animal activity groups in the 48 contiguous states and Alaska. In addition, five other focus areas were identified for this study: 1) public attitudes toward critical wildlife and natural habitat issues (e.g., endangered species, predator control, hunting, trapping

*Supported by grant #1416000977056 from the United States Fish and Wildlife Service, Department of the Interior.

†Reprinted from *International Journal for the Study of Animal Problems* 1(2)1980.

and habitat preservation); 2) the size and social characteristics of various wildlife and domestic animal activity groups (e.g., hunters, birdwatchers, pet owners, and humane and wildlife protection organization members); 3) public knowledge of animals and species preferences; 4) historical trends in uses and perception of animals during the twentieth century; and 5) children's knowledge of, and attitudes and behavior toward animals.

This report will review some of the results of this investigation. Space limitations, however, restrict the amount of information that can be covered and, thus, some data will be omitted and others only cursorily examined. No data will be provided on the historical or children's studies as these investigations are still in progress.

The results presented in this paper are largely based on a national survey of 3,107 randomly selected Americans in the 48 contiguous states and Alaska. A special oversampling was drawn in the Rocky Mountain States and Alaska in order to ensure sufficient numbers in these important regions. In all analyses referring to the entire American population, however, this oversampling was accounted for, resulting in a total national sample size of 2,455. Respondents were chosen according to a probability random selection method roughly ensuring that every individual in the American population had an equal chance of being selected. In addition, a minimum of one initial contact and three call-backs were included before the designated respondent could be dropped. These methods considerably enhanced the representativeness of the sample. Each respondent was personally interviewed for approximately sixty minutes. Twenty-two percent of those contacted refused an interview, thirteen percent could not be located after the fourth interview attempt, and approximately four percent terminated the interview before its completion. In spite of these limitations, a comparison with the national census suggested that the sample was a relatively good cross section of the American population with a slightly higher socioeconomic profile (age, sex and race differences were nonsignificant). In addition to the national sample, special mail surveys, using the same questionnaire, were conducted with members of the National Cattlemen's, American Sheep Producer's and National Trappers' Associations, as well as with subscribers to the magazine, *Vegetarian Times*.

Five pretests were conducted to develop reliable and valid attitude questions. Attitude scales were developed based on a typology of nine basic attitudes toward animals. Cluster and other multivariate analyses were employed in the scale construction process. No useful scale was devised to measure the *aesthetic* attitude. Additionally, a *neutralistic* attitude scale could not be usefully distinguished from a *negativistic* scale and, thus, only one scale was developed including elements of both the *negativistic* and *neutralistic* attitudes, with perhaps more of the latter. Sixty-five attitude questions were used in the development of these scales, with the smallest scale (*ecologistic*) consisting of four questions and the largest (*utilitarian*) thirteen. Where appropriate, the strength of the response (e.g., strongly versus slightly agree/disagree) was included. Scale scores ranged from 0 to 11 for the *ecologistic* attitude scale, and from 0 to 27 for the *utilitarian* attitude scale. The independence of the resulting eight attitude scales was suggested by relatively small scale intercorrelations—14 under .20; the smallest, .04; the largest negative correlation, −.42 (the *naturalistic* and *negativistic* attitudes); and the largest positive correlation, .40 (the *naturalistic* and *ecologistic*).

In addition, more than 500 indices were reviewed and three pretests conducted to develop a "knowledge of animals" scale. The resulting 33-item true-false and multiple choice knowledge scale covered all vertebrate classes, and five questions dealt with invertebrates. All questions were omitted which favored specialized knowledge on the part of any particular animal activity group. The distribution of knowledge scale scores was roughly normal, with a mean of 52.8 on a range of 0 to 100.

ATTITUDES TOWARD ANIMALS

As previously indicated, prior research identified a typology of basic attitudes toward animals. As this typology is described in detail elsewhere, only crude, one-sentence definitions are provided below (Kellert 1976; Kellert 1979b).

Naturalistic—Primary interest in and affection for wildlife and the outdoors.

Ecologistic—Primary concern for the environment as a system, for interrelationships between wildlife species and natural habitats.

Humanistic—Primary interest in and strong affection for individual animals, principally pets.

Moralistic—Primary concern for the right and wrong treatment of animals, with strong opposition to exploitation of and cruelty toward animals.

Scientistic—Primary interest in the physical attributes and biological functioning of animals.

Aesthetic—Primary interest in the artistic and symbolic characteristics of animals.

Utilitarian—Primary concern for the practical and material value of animals.

Dominionistic—Primary satisfactions derived from mastery and control over animals, typically in sporting situations.

Negativistic—Primary orientation an active avoidance of animals due to dislike or fear.

Neutralistic—Primary orientation a passive avoidance of animals due to indifference and lack of interest.

The scales used in the national survey are crude approximations of the attitude types and only in the broadest sense measure their true prevalence and distribution in the American population. Nevertheless, the relative frequency of the attitudes in the national sample was assessed by standardizing the various scale scores on a 0 to 1 range, plotting a regression line through the scale score distribution frequencies for each attitude, and using these frequency curves and regression figures to estimate the comparative "popularity" of the attitudes. As particular scores on one attitude scale cannot be equated with similar scores on other scales, this procedure only roughly indicates the relative frequency of the eight attitudes in the American population. The results of this analysis are presented in Figure 1.

These results suggest that the most common attitudes toward animals in contemporary American society, by a large margin, are the *humanistic, moralistic, utilitarian, and negativistic* attitudes. In many respects, these attitudes can be subsumed under two broad and conflicting dimensional perceptions of animals. The *moralistic* and *utilitarian* attitudes clash around the theme of human exploitation of animals. The former opposes many exploitative uses of animals involving death and presumed suffering (e.g., hunting, trapping, whaling and laboratory experimentation), while the latter endorses such utilization, or other human activities which might adversely affect animals, if significant human material benefits result. In a somewhat analogous fashion, the *negativistic* and *humanistic* attitudes tend to clash, although in a more latent fashion, around the theme of affection for animals. The former is characterized by indifference and incredulity toward the notion of "loving" animals, while the latter involves intense emotional attachments to animals. The relative popularity of these four attitudes in contemporary American society may suggest a dynamic basis for the conflict and misunderstanding often existing today over issues involving people and animals.

The *scientistic* and *dominionistic* attitudes, according to the results of Figure 1, are the least common perceptions of animals among the American public. The shape of the *naturalistic* frequency curve suggests that this attitude is strongly present among a minority of Americans, but relatively weakly evident among the majority. The *ecologistic* scale score distribution indicates a substantial number of respondents expressing modest support for this viewpoint, but very

Figure 1
ATTITUDE DISTRIBUTION CURVES: ENTIRE POPULATION

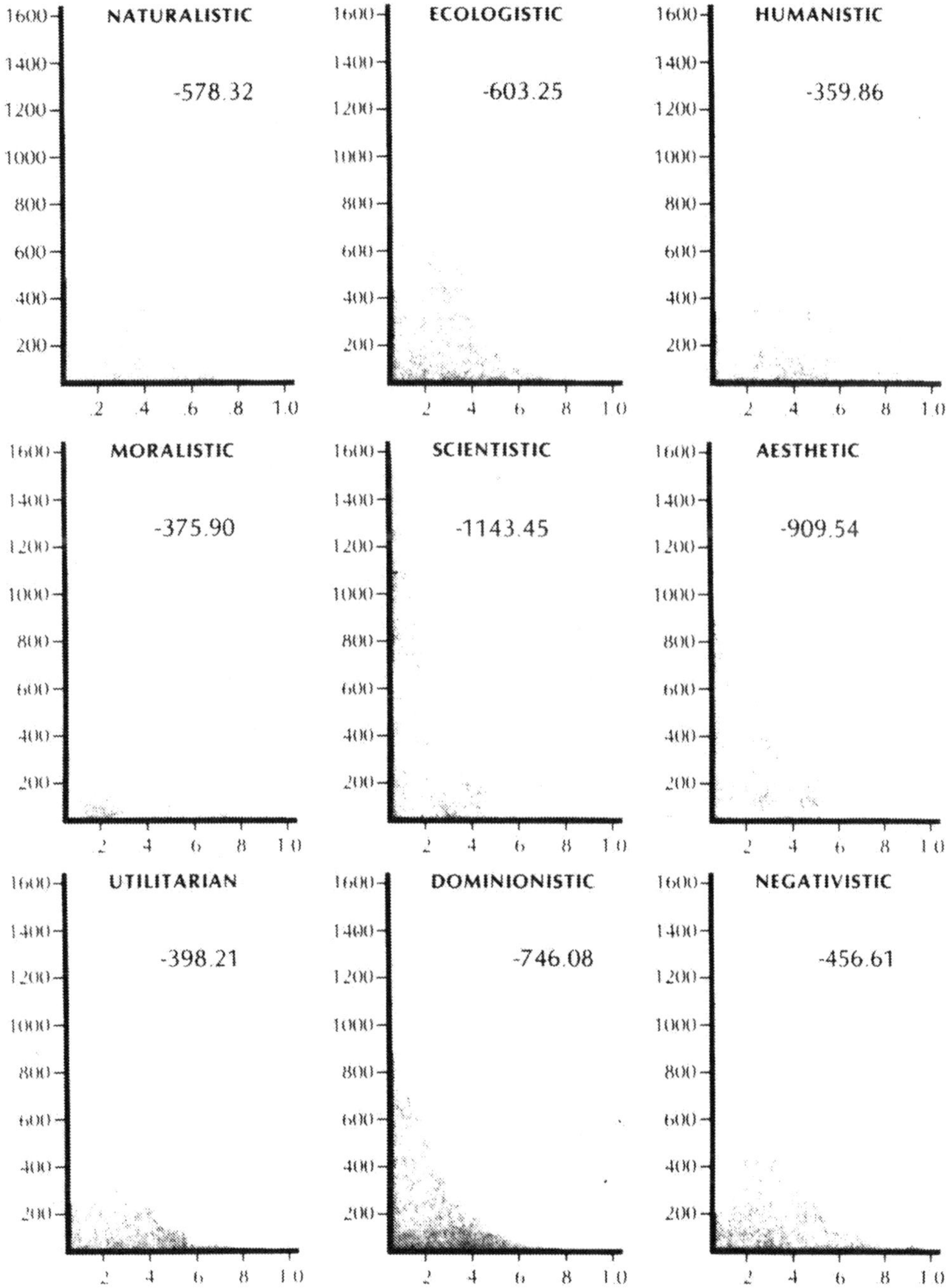

Vertical Axis: No. of People Horizontal Axis: Score

Figure 2
EDUCATION GROUPS BY SELECTED KNOWLEDGE AND ATTITUDE SCALES

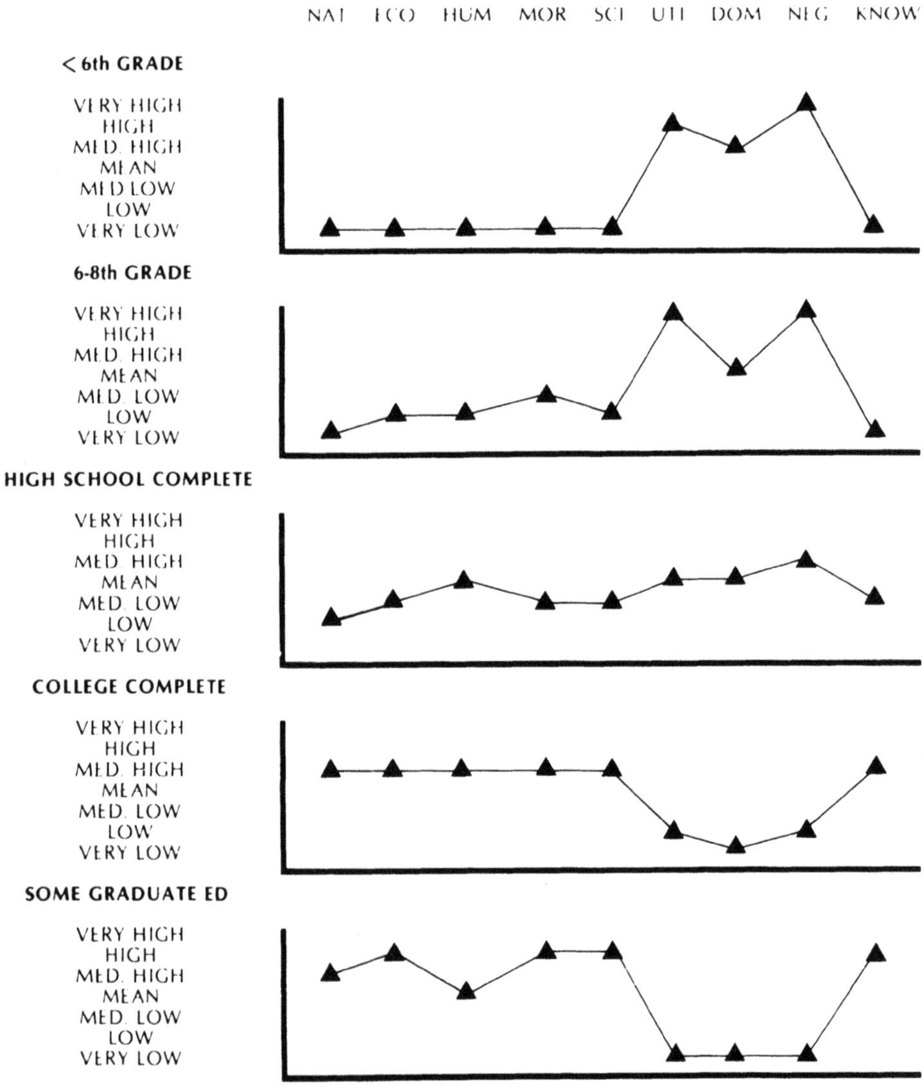

Figure 3
REGIONS BY SELECTED KNOWLEDGE AND ATTITUDE SCALES

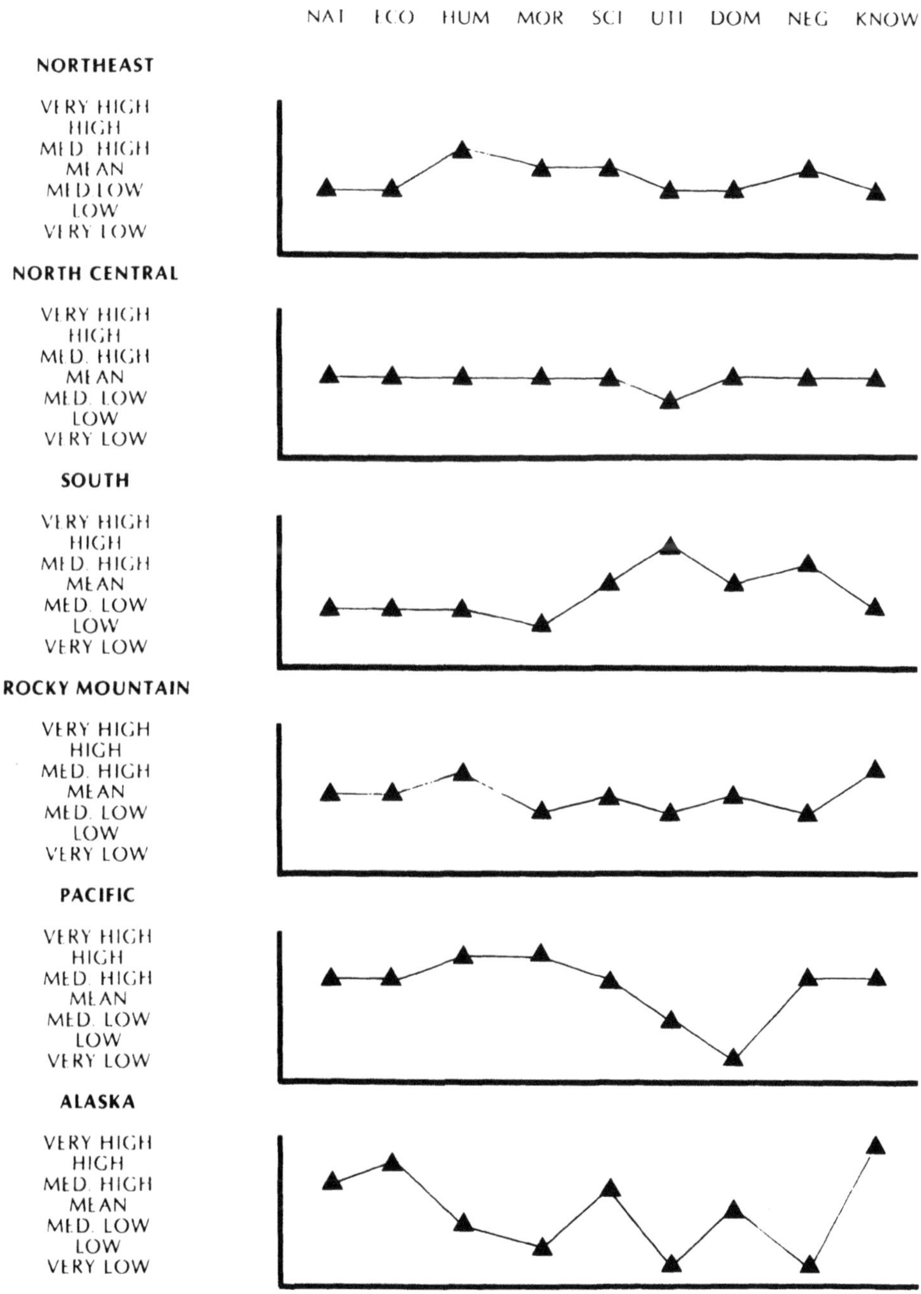

Figure 4

AGE GROUPS BY SELECTED KNOWLEDGE AND ATTITUDE SCALES

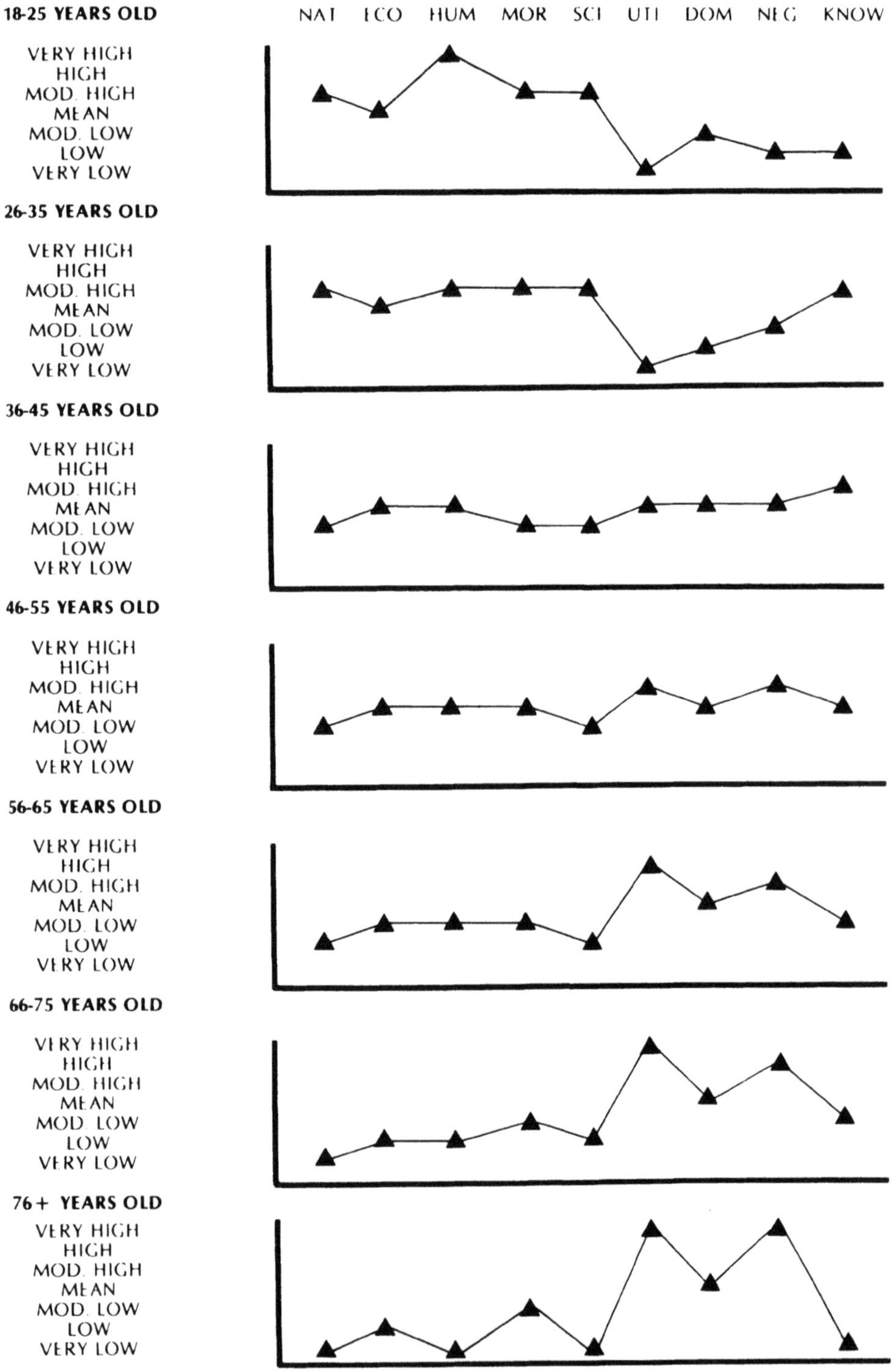

Figure 5

RACE GROUPS BY SELECTED KNOWLEDGE AND ATTITUDE SCALES

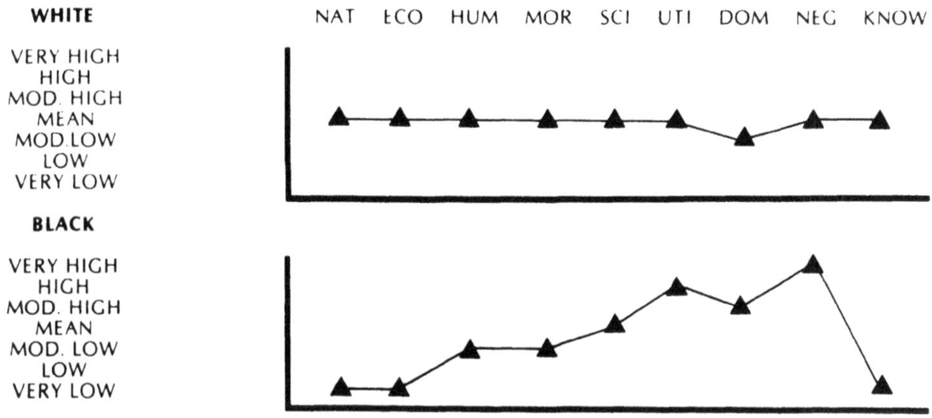

few strongly oriented in this fashion. Impressions on the percentage distribution of the attitudes in the American public, their most common behavioral expressions, and benefits or values generally associated with each attitude type are summarized in Table 1.

The distribution of the attitudes among various demographic groups (e.g., age, sex, urban-rural residence and income) and animal activity groups (e.g., hunters, birders and organization members) was also examined. These attitude distributions are reviewed in terms of relative frequencies on a single attitude, and by comparisons of one or more groups across all the attitude types. The first type of analysis is presented in Tables I through V, while the second type is included in Figures 2-5. In order to expedite the discussion, only the *naturalistic, humanistic, moralistic, utilitarian, dominionistic,* and *negativistic* attitude results are described, although tabular results are provided for the other attitude types.

THE NATURALISTIC ATTITUDE

A comparison of *naturalistic* attitude scale means among various animal activity groups (Table I) reveals that nature "hunters" had the highest scores, along with environmental protection organization members (e.g., members of the Sierra Club, Wilderness Society) and birders. The *naturalistic* scores of nature hunters were far higher than those of meat or recreation hunters. Anti-hunters, livestock raisers, and fishermen had comparatively low scores on this attitude scale, although all animal activity groups had higher mean scores on the *na-*

turalistic scale than did the general population.

Among social demographic groups (Table II) Alaskans had the highest *naturalistic* scores. Other social groups with high *naturalistic* scale scores included the college-educated, the affluent, professionals, persons under 35, respondents from moderate-sized population areas, Pacific Coast residents, and those who rarely or never attended religious services. In contrast, the poorly educated, nonwhites, the elderly, low income respondents, and persons of farm background scored substantially below the general population average on this dimension.

The possibility that variable differences were a function of interrelationships among certain demographic factors prompted the use of a statistical procedure, analysis of variance. Basically, this test examined the combined effect of a number of demographic groups on the attitude scales. When the following factors were subjected to analysis of variance—age, sex, race, marital status, occupation, education, income, region, population of present residence, and attendance at religious services—marital status, occupation and population of residence were not found to be significantly related to the *naturalistic* scale.

Multiple classification analysis is a statistical technique based on analysis of variance which allows one to determine which categories of a variable contribute most to the overall significance of the variable—e.g., which specific regional or educational groups are most related to the *naturalistic* scale after all other demographic variables have been taken into account. According to the results of this analysis, (Tables III and IV), the most *naturalistic* groups were graduate school and college education, Alaskan and Pacific Coast residents, respondents under 35 years of age, and persons who rarely or never attended religious service. In contrast, the least *naturalistic* were blacks, respondents with less than a high school education, and persons over 56 years of age.

THE HUMANISTIC ATTITUDE

Among animal activity groups, humane and environmental protection organization members, zoo visitors, anti-hunters, and scientific study hobbyists scored very high on the *humanistic* scale (Table I). In contrast, livestock producers, nature hunters, and surprisingly, birdwatchers had much lower scores. Apparently these latter groups, in light of their high scores on the *naturalistic* scale (with the exception of livestock producers), were far more oriented toward wildlife and outdoor recreation values than toward the benefits derived from love of animals, particularly pets.

Persons under 25 years of age, those earning between $20-35,000, females, respondents who rarely or never attended religious services, and Pacific Coast residents were the most *humanistically*-oriented demographic groups (Tables II-IV). In contrast, farmers, persons over 76 years of age, residents of the most rural areas, and males had the lowest scores on this attitude dimension. Analysis of variance results suggested that size of town, education, marital status and race were not significantly related.

THE MORALISTIC ATTITUDE

Those demographic groups expressing the greatest *moralistic* concern were Pacific Coast residents, the highly educated, those engaged in clerical occupations, females, persons who rarely or never attended religious services, and respondents under 35 years of age (Tables II-IV). Groups least troubled by animal welfare and cruelty issues were rural residents, farmers, respondents from Alaska and the South, and males.

Animal activity groups scoring high on the *moralistic* scale (Table I) included humane and environmental protection organization members and anti-hunters. Scientific study hobbyists also had high scores on this dimension. Recreation and meat hunters, sportsmen organization members, trappers, fishermen, and livestock producers scored very low on this attitude scale.

THE UTILITARIAN ATTITUDE

Farmers, the elderly, blacks and Southern respondents had the highest scores on the *utilitarian* scale. In contrast, persons under 35 years of age, those with graduate school education, Alaska respondents, single persons and residents of areas of one million or more population indicated the least *utilitarian* interest in animals (Tables II, III and IV). Among animal activity groups, livestock producers, meat hunters and fishermen displayed an especially strong *utilitarian* orientation in contrast to members of humane, wildlife protection and environmental protection organizations, and, to a somewhat lesser degree, scientific study hobbyists, backpackers, and birdwatchers (Table I).

THE DOMINIONISTIC ATTITUDE

The most *dominionistically*-oriented animal activity groups were trappers and all three types of hunters. Humane organization members and anti-hunters had the lowest scores on this attitude scale, suggesting that differences in *dominionistic* perception of animals represented a basic and important distinction in the perspectives of hunters and anti-hunters. Zoo visitors and environmental protection organization members also had comparatively low scores on this scale (Table I).

Farmers, males, Alaska and Rocky Mountain residents, blacks and those with high incomes were the most *dominionistically*-oriented demographic groups. Females, Pacific Coast respondents, the highly educated, clerical workers, and persons rarely or never attending religious services scored lowest on this scale (Tables II, III and V). Differences among the most affluent and educated on the *dominionistic* scale were in marked contrast to similarities between these higher socioeconomic groups on other attitude scales, and suggested that high income and advanced education do not necessarily result in the same perceptions of animals.

THE NEGATIVISTIC ATTITUDE

No animal activity group revealed marked disinterest or dislike of animals, as measured by the *negativistic* attitude scale (Table I) although livestock producers did score only slightly above the general population mean. Interestingly, anti-hunters had comparatively high scores on this dimension, suggesting that broad principles concerning the ethical treatment of animals were more salient considerations in opposition to hunting than general interest in animals. Environmental and wildlife protection organization members, scientific study hobbyists, and birdwatchers were the least *negativistic*. Among demographic groups, the elderly, those of limited education and females had the highest *negativistic* scale scores. In contrast, persons with graduate school education, Alaska residents, respondents under 25 years of age, and those residing in areas under 500 population were the least *negativistic* in their perception of animals (Tables II, III and V). *Ecologistic* and *scientistic* attitude scale differences are indicated in Tables I-V.

ADDITIONAL FINDINGS

Attitude profiles of selected demographic groups are provided as an illustration of comparative group variations across all of the attitude dimensions. Educational group differences (Figure 2), for example, indicate that respondents of limited education had considerably lower scores than the highly educated on all the attitude dimensions with the exception of the *dominionistic, utilitarian* and *negativistic* scales. These findings suggest a relative disinterest in and lack of affection for animals among the least educated, with the possible exception of situations involving sporting satisfactions and material gain. Indeed, the dramatically evident differences among the education groups pointed to a fundamental divergence in the perceptions of animals and the natural world among various socioeconomic groups in our society.

Regional differences (Figure 3) were also fairly large and somewhat surprising. One of the most striking results was the stronger wildlife interest, concern and appreciation of Alaska respondents. In general, the western states revealed greater wildlife appreciaton and knowledge while the South was characterized by the least interest and concern for animals and the most *utilitarian* orientation.

Age and race profiles are presented in Figures 4 and 5. Differences between the very oldest and youngest respondents were especially striking on nearly every attitude dimension, particularly on the *naturalistic, humanistic* and *utilitarian* scales. Those over 75 and 25 years of age were only similar in their relative lack of knowledge of animals. Race results suggested a comparative lack of interest in, and concern and affection for animals among nonwhites.

KNOWLEDGE OF ANIMALS

All animal activity groups scored significantly higher on the knowledge of animals scale than did the general public (Table 2). However, birdwatchers, nature hunters, scientific study hobbyists and all types of conservation-related organization members had significantly higher scores than did livestock producers, anti-hunters, zoo enthusiasts, sport and recreation hunters and fishermen. Among demographic groups (Tables 2 and 3), the most knowledgeable were persons with higher education (especially graduate training), Alaska and Rocky Mountain residents, males and respondents who rarely or never attended religious services. In contrast, the least informed about animals—even after accounting for the interrelationships of all demographic variables—were blacks, respondents with less than a high school education, persons over 75 and, interestingly, under 25 years of age, and residents of cities of one million or more population.

The American public, as a whole, was characterized by extremely limited knowledge of animals. For example, on four questions dealing with endangered species (Table 4), no more than one-third of the respondents obtained the correct answer—only 26 percent knew the manatee is not an insect and just 24 percent correctly answered the statement, "timber wolves, bald eagles and coyotes are all endangered species of animals." Regarding other knowledge questions, just 13 percent knew that raptors are not small rodents and one-half of the sample incorrectly answered the statement, "spiders have ten legs." A better but still distressingly low 54 percent knew that veal does not come from lamb, and just 57 percent indicated the correct answer to the question, "most insects have backbones." The knowledge questions were divided into a number of generic categories, and a comparison of mean scores revealed that the public was most knowledgeable on questions concerning animals implicated in human injury, pets, basic characteristics of animals (e.g., "all adult birds have feathers") and domestic animals in general. On the other hand, they were least knowledgeable about invertebrates, "taxonomic" distinctions (e.g., "Koala bears are not really bears") and predators. The respective mean scores for these categories were:

	Mean Knowledge Score
Animals That Inflict Human Injury	63.4
Pets	55.6
Basic Biological Characteristics	55.3
Domestic Animals Other Than Pets	53.4
Predators	47.1
Taxonomic Distinctions	39.8
Invertebrates	36.6
Overall Mean for 33 Question Knowledge Scale with 0 to 100 Scoring Range	52.8

The general public was also questioned on its perceived familiarity with or awareness of eight relatively prominent wildlife issues (Table 5). The three most widely recognized issues were the killing of baby seals for their fur (43 percent knowledgeable), the effects of pesticides such as DDT on birds (42 percent knowledgeable), and the use of steel leghold traps to trap wild animals (38 percent knowledgeable). The least familiar issues included the use of steel versus lead shot by waterfowl hunters (14 percent knowledgeable) and the Tennessee Valley Authority/Tellico Dam/Snail Darter controversy (17 percent knowledgeable). The public appeared to be far more aware of relatively emotional issues involving specific, attractive and typically large and "higher" animals, compared to issues of a more abstract nature, involving indirect impacts on wildlife due to habitat loss, and dealing with "lower" animals.

SPECIES PREFERENCE

The national sample was queried on its feelings about 33 species ranked on a seven point like/dislike scale (the most and least liked are indicated in Table 6). The most preferred were two common domestic animals—the dog and the horse—followed by two familiar and highly aesthetic bird species and one insect order—the robin, swan and butterfly. The trout—a popular and highly attractive game species—was the best-liked fish, and the most preferred wild predator was the eagle. The most favored wild mammalian species was the elephant.

On the other hand, three of the four least-liked animals were biting, stinging invertebrates—the cockroach, mosquito and wasp. The third, fifth and sixth least preferred animals—the rat, rattlesnake and bat—have all been implicated in physical injury or disease inflicted on human beings. Relatively negative views of the coyote and wolf were interesting to note given the prevailing controversy over predator control programs in the United States and the considerable amount of favorable publicity received by the wolf in recent years. High standard deviation scores for the wolf, coyote, lizard, skunk, vulture, bat, shark, and cat suggested considerable variation in public opinion regarding the positive and negative qualities of these animals.

A qualitative assessment of the most and least preferred animals, as well as a categorical mean grouping of the 33 animals according to particular qualities (e.g., attractive, unattractive, predator, etc.—see Table 6), suggested a number of particularly important factors in public preference for different species. These factors included:

1. Size (usually, the larger the animal, the more preferred)
2. Aesthetics
3. Intelligence (not only capacity for reason but also for feeling and emotion)
4. Dangerous to Humans
5. Likelihood of Inflicting Property Damage
6. Predatory Tendencies
7. Phylogenetic Relatedness to Humans
8. Cultural and Historical Relationship
9. Relationship to Human Society: pet, domestic farm, game, pest, native wildlife, exotic wildlife
10. Texture (generally, the more unfamiliar to humans, the less preferred)
11. Mode of Locomotion (generally, the more unfamiliar to humans, the less preferred)
12. Economic Value of the Species

CRITICAL WILDLIFE ISSUES

Public attitudes toward over thirty critical wildlife and natural habitat issues were explored. Insufficient space precludes a review of all these findings, and a detailed description can be found elsewhere (Kellert 1979a). Only a brief summary of results pertaining to the following issues will be provided here: endangered species, predator control, hunting, trapping, harvesting of selected marine mammals and wildlife habitat protection.

Endangered Species

Protection of endangered species was generally explored in the context of various socioeconomic impacts including energy development, water use, forest utilization, and industrial development. The results graphically depicted in Table 7 concern the situation of costly modification of an energy development project in order to protect varying kinds of endangered species. While the public overwhelmingly accepted this sacrifice to protect species of eagle, mountain lion, trout, crocodile and butterfly, less than a majority were willing to tolerate this socioeconomic impact for the sake of plant, snake or spider species.

The results of Table 8 deal with a Tellico Dam–type question involving the protection of a threatened, unknown fish species at the cost of forfeiting various needs derived from these water uses— hydroelectric energy, increased drinking supplies and agricultural irrigation—the public strongly disapproved of curtailing the water projects to protect the unknown fish species. On the other hand, in situations entailing relatively "nonessential" benefits—water for cooling industrial machinery and to make a lake for recreational purposes—less than a majority approved of the projects.

The results in Table 9 cover two additional endangered species questions. The first concerns the preservation of large amounts of wilderness habitat to protect the grizzly bear at the expense of forest products and jobs. The results suggest a moderate, but significant public willingness to accept this economic sacrifice to protect the species. The second question concerns the filling of wetlands to build an industrial plant in an area of high unemployment. The endangered species is an unspecified bird species and, in line with the grizzly bear result, the public indicated a significant but moderate support for protection despite the socioeconomic impact.

These results and related literature suggest eight factors critically related to the public's willingness to protect endangered wildlife (Ehrenfeld 1970; Guggisberg 1970; Ziswiler 1967). The first is aesthetics, which was probably relevant in results involving the butterfly, snake and spider. The second is phylogenetic relatedness to humans. Generally speaking, the closer the biological relation of the endangered animal to human beings, the greater the likelihood of public support for the species. The third factor is the reason for endangerment, with typically greater public sympathy in cases involving direct causes of endangerment (e.g., overexploitation or persecution) than in situations involving indirect impacts (e.g., habitat loss due to expanding human populations). The fourth factor is the economic value of the species being exploited. The fifth concerns the numbers and types of people affected by efforts to protect the endangered animal. The cultural and historical significance of the endangered species is the sixth factor, and may have been involved in public sympathy for the bald eagle and trout. The seventh variable is the public's knowledge and familiarity with the endangered animal. Public support for the American crocodile may reflect this factor. Finally, the perceived humaneness of the activity threatening the species may be important. For example, the relatively slight opposition to water uses endangering an unknown fish species may have stemmed partially from assumptions regarding the capacities of fish to suffer or experience pain.

The willingness to protect endangered wildlife varied considerably among diverse demographic groups. These variations are summarized in the results of an endangered species protection scale developed on the basis of the four previously described endangered species questions. As Table 10 indicates, significantly higher scores (i.e., a greater willingness to protect endangered species) were found among the highly educated, younger and single respondents, persons residing in areas of more than one million population, and residents of Alaska. In contrast, older respondents, persons with less than an eighth grade education, farmers, residents of highly rural areas and residents of the South had significantly lower endangered species protection scores.

One of the most controversial issues facing the wildlife field today is predator control. Table 11 deals with the issue of controlling coyotes that prey on domestic livestock. Five control options were considered and the views of an informed and uninformed general public, as well as members of the American Sheep Producers and National Cattlemen's Associations were contrasted.* Options considered included the two most controversial control strategies: indiscriminate population reductions by shooting or trapping as many coyotes as possible, and poison-

*Results of the fifth option—compensating ranchers for livestock losses out of general tax revenues—is not presented. Both the general public and livestock producers were opposed to this alternative.

ing. The public was moderately opposed to indiscriminate population reductions (with the informed public significantly more opposed) and overwhelmingly against the use of poisons (even though this alternative was described as the least expensive). In dramatic contrast, livestock producers were strongly in favor of both control strategies (indeed, these differences were, statistically, the largest found in the study).

As indicated in Table 11, nearly 79 percent of the public supported the notion of hunting only individual coyotes known to have killed livestock. Additionally, more than two-thirds approved of capturing and relocating coyotes in areas away from livestock despite this being described as a very expensive solution. While livestock producers were strongly opposed to coyote relocation efforts, they were somewhat divided on the notion of hunting only individual coyotes responsible for livestock loss.

In general, the predator control results indicated a strong public concern for the humaneness and specificity of the control method as indicated by strong opposition to the use of poisons and support for controlling only individual offender coyotes.

An equally controversial issue is the public's attitude toward hunting. Attitudes toward six different kinds of hunting were explored. Table 12 indicates the public overwhelmingly approved of the two most pragmatically justified types of hunting—subsistence hunting as practiced by traditional native Americans and hunting exclusively for meat regardless of the identity of the hunter. On the other hand, approximately 60 percent opposed hunting solely for recreational or sporting purposes, whether for waterfowl or big game. Moreover, over 80 percent objected to the notion of hunting for a trophy. Perhaps most interestingly, 64 percent approved of hunting for recreational purposes if this also included using the meat. The implication is that hunting is viewed as too serious an activity to be engaged in solely for its sporting or recreational value, but is acceptable if the animal's meat is to be consumed.

Over 70 percent of the public objected to the use of the steel leghold trap. No difference was found between knowledgeable and uninformed people. On the other hand, nearly all trappers saw nothing wrong with the use of these traps (Table 13).

Somewhat unexpectedly, 77 percent of the general public approved of killing whales for a useful product so long as the species was not endangered. A very different perception of the dolphin was indicated with nearly 70 percent willing to pay a higher price for tuna if this resulted in fishermen killing fewer porpoises in their nets. The disparity between these two marine mammal findings may have been related to the colorful and romantic history of whaling in America, as opposed to the absence of any tradition in this country of harvesting porpoises.

On a variety of wildlife habitat protection questions, the public indicated a moderate but significant willingness to protect wildlife habitat even at the expense of various human benefits. The results of four habitat protection questions are indicated in Table 14. In each situation, a trade-off was proposed, placing the protection of wildlife habitat in the context of various socioeconomic costs. In order to maintain waterfowl habitat, the filling of wetlands for housing development is sacrificed; to protect rangeland from overgrazing, higher beef prices result. The wilderness, housing development, and livestock grazing findings were remarkably similar—a moderate but significant majority of the public was willing to protect wildlife habitat even at the expense of the stated human benefits. Seventy-six percent favored the harvesting of timber in ways which helped wildlife even if this resulted in increased lumber prices.

CONCLUSION

A variety of results have been presented suggesting considerable public interest in and affection for animals and a willingness to support wildlife conservation in this country. On the other hand, a great deal of variation and conflict was found in the attitudes, perceptions and knowledge of animals among diverse groups in American society. While a bedrock of affection and concern was found, it appears that much needs to happen before this appreciative orientation is usefully broadened to encompass a more biologically knowledgeable and ethically sensitive feeling for animals. Those responsible for animal welfare and natural environments should recognize this public sympathy and interest in animals and devote increasing efforts to addressing the needs for greater awareness and understanding. The challenges are great for wildlife professionals, humane educators, natural resource managers, and others responsible for the future well-being of the nonhuman world. Until these human factors are more properly understood, however, it is doubtful that the continued erosion of land resources and destruction of fauna will be arrested.

Table 1. Attitude Occurrence in American Society

Attitude	Estimated % Of American Population Strongly Oriented Toward The Attitude†	Common Behavioral Expressions	Most Related Values/Benefits
Naturalistic	10	Outdoor wildlife related recreation — Backcountry use, nature birding and nature hunting	Outdoor recreation
Ecologistic	7	Conservation support, activism and membership, ecological study	Ecological
Humanistic	35	Pets, wildlife tourism, casual zoo visitation	Companionship, affection
Moralistic	20	Animal welfare support/membership, kindness to animals	Ethical, existence
Scientistic	1	Scientific study/hobbies, collecting	Scientific
Aesthetic	15	Nature appreciation, art, wildlife tourism	Aesthetic
Utilitarian	20	Consumption of furs, raising meat, bounties, meat hunting	Consumptive, utilitarian
Dominionistic	3	Animal spectator sports, trophy hunting	Sporting
Negativistic	2	Cruelty, overt fear behavior	Little or negative
Neutralistic	35	Avoidance of animal behavior	Little or negative

†Totals more than 100% as persons can be strongly oriented toward more than one attitude

Table 2. Animal Knowledge Scale by Selected Groups: 1978 National Sample Maximum Score = 100

Animal Activity Groups

Group	Score
Birdwatchers	68.3
Wildlf. Protect. Org. Memb.	65.6
Nature Hunters	65.3
Scientific Study	65.0
Env. Protect. Org. Member	64.4
Humane Org. Memb.	62.8
Sportsmen Org. Memb.	62.7
Gen. Conserv. Org.Memb.	62.5
Backpackers	57.5
Meat Hunters	57.4
Fishermen	56.4
Sport/Rec. Hunters	56.3
Zoo Visitors	54.8
Livestock Raisers	53.9
Anti-Hunters	53.9
General Population	52.9

Selected Demographic Groups

Group	Score
Ph.D.	67.7
Non-Ph.D. Graduate	61.6
Alaska	60.6
Law or Medical Degree	60.4
College Complete	56.8
Rocky Mountain Region	56.8
$50,000-99,999 Income	56.7
Professional	56.6
Some College	56.3
25,000-49,999 Pop. Childhood	55.7
General Population	52.9
<$5,000 Income	49.3
Widowed	49.1
6th-8th Grade Education	47.8
Black	46.1
75+ Years Old	46.0
<6th Grade Education	44.4

1978 Mail Sample

Group	Score
Natl. Trappers	66.0
Cattlement	63.5
Sheep Producers	61.8

Table 3. Animal Knowledge Scale Analysis of Variance and Multiple Classification Analysis Results Against Selected Demographic Variables

Analysis of Variance

	F Value
Age	7.67‡
Population of Present Residence	3.09‡
Region	5.93‡
Education	31.83‡
Occupation	0.23
Religiosity	4.75‡
Income	5.31‡
Marital Status	3.07†
Race	30.31‡
Sex	66.82‡

Multiple Classification Analysis: Largest Positive and Negative Deviations After Adjusting for Independent and Covariant Variables

Graduate Education	7.73
Alaska	4.86
Rocky Mountain States	2.75
College Education	2.36
Male	2.18
Rarely/Never Attend Religious Services	1.96
1 Million+ Population	-2.07
18-25 Years Old	-2.30
76+ Years Old	-3.12
9th-11th Grade Education	-3.36
Less than 8th Grade Education	-5.10
Black	-5.50

†Significance ≤ 0.05
‡Significance ≤ 0.01

Table 4. Knowledge of Endangered Species

Question or Statement	% Correct Answer	% Wrong Answer	% Don't Know
The passenger pigeon and the Carolina parakeet are now extinct.	26.2	23.1	50.6
Pesticides were a major factor in the decline of brown pelicans.	33.3	9.9	56.8
The manatee is an insect.	25.6	23.1	51.3
Timber wolves, bald eagles, and coyotes are all endangered species of animals.	25.6	61.7	13.8

Table 5. Awareness of Selected Wildlife Issues†

Issue	% Knowledgeable	% Not Knowledgeable
Killing baby seals for their fur	43	32
Effects of pesticides such as DDT on birds	42	32
Using steel leghold traps to trap wild animals	38	37
Endangered Species Act	34	40
Killing of livestock by coyotes	23	52
Tuna-porpoise controversy	27	55
Tennessee Valley Authority Tellico Dam/snail darter issue	17	70
Use of steel shot versus lead shot by waterfowl hunters	14	75

†The *knowledgeable* category combines the groups of very and moderately knowledgeable, the *not knowledgeable* category combines the groups of very little and no knowledge. The *slightly knowledgeable* category results are omitted in this comparison.

Table 6. Animal Preference Means

Most Liked Animals		Least Liked Animals		Species Preference Mean/Scores For Selected Animal Categories	
Animal	X Value†	Animal	X Value†	Animal	Mean Score†
Dog	1.70	Cockroach	6.45	Domestic animals	2.08
Horse	1.79	Mosquito	6.27	Attractive animals	2.38
Swan	1.97	Rat	6.26	Game animals	2.59
Robin	1.99	Wasp	5.68	Birds	2.98
Butterfly	2.04	Rattlesnake	5.66	Mammals	3.40
Trout	2.12	Bat	5.35	Amphibians, reptiles, fish	3.55
Salmon	2.26	Vulture	4.91	Predators	3.91
Eagle	2.29	Shark	4.82	Animals known to cause human property damage	4.02
Elephant	2.63	Skunk	4.42	Invertebrates	4.64
Turtle	2.69	Lizard	4.13	Animals known to inflict human injury	5.08
Cat	2.74	Crow	4.06	Unattractive animals	5.46
Ladybug	2.78	Coyote	4.02	Biting and stinging invertebrates	6.13
Raccoon	2.80	Wolf	3.98		

†Lower score indicates greater preference

Table 7. Public Attitudes Regarding Changing of an Energy Project to Protect Endangered Species Types

Question: A recent law passed to protect endangered species may result in changing some energy development projects at greater cost. As a result, it has been suggested that endangered species protection be limited only to certain animals and plants. Which of the following endangered species would you favor protecting, *even if it resulted in higher costs for an energy development project?*

		% Favor			% Oppose				
Species	**# Polled**	**Strong**	**Moderate**	**Slight**	**Slight**	**Moderate**	**Strong**	**No Opinion**	**% Favor Overall**
Butterfly (Silverspot)	2452	9.5	29.2	25.0	9.3	15.1	3.7	8.2	64
Mountain Lion	2453	16.7	35.9	20.6	6.6	11.9	2.8	5.6	73
Fish (Agassiz Trout)	2450	11.9	36.7	22.4	7.2	10.7	2.6	8.2	71
Spider (Kauai Wolf)	2452	4.7	11.9	17.4	13.8	28.9	14.0	9.2	34
American Crocodile	2452	13.2	35.0	21.5	7.3	13.5	4.2	5.2	70
Furbish Lousewort	2451	5.7	20.8	21.1	10.8	17.8	5.2	18.4	48
Eastern Indigo Snake	2452	6.0	19.2	18.2	10.7	25.3	12.4	8.0	43
Bald Eagle	2452	43.9	37.0	8.1	2.6	4.3	1.2	2.8	89

Table 8. Public Attitudes in Regard to Various Water Uses If Such Use Would Endanger a Fish Species

Statement: Various kinds of fish have been threatened with extinction because of dams, canals and other water projects. Please indicate if you would approve of the following water uses if they were to endanger a species of fish.

Water Use	# Polled	% Approve Strong	% Approve Moderate	% Approve Slight	% Disapprove Slight	% Disapprove Moderate	% Disapprove Strong
A. Cool industrial machinery†	2316	3.1	21.7 (48)‡	23.2	17.1	22.1 (46)	7.1
B. Provide hydroelectric power	2336	7.7	38.2 (72)	25.7	10.2	10.1 (24)	3.3
C. Increase human drinking supplies	2391	18.6	51.6 (87)	16.5	4.9	4.2 (11)	1.6
D. Dammed for recreational use	2374	3.6	17.6 (39)	18.1	15.5	28.6 (57)	13.3
E. Diverted for agricultural irrigation	2384	12.7	47.1 (83)	23.4	6.8	5.2 (14)	1.9

†Difference between approve and disapprove on this is not significant ($Z = 0.75$, $P = 0.45$)

Differences on B - E are highly significant ($P < 0.0001$)

‡Numbers in parentheses ( ) are totals approving or disapproving

Table 9. General Public Attitudes toward Protection of Forest Land and Wetlands for Endangered Species

Question	% Agree	% Disagree	Z Value
It has been suggested that 5 million acres of national forest land be set aside so that the endangered grizzly bear remain undisturbed. The timber industry objects, saying that jobs and needed lumber will be lost. Would you agree to protect the endangered grizzly bear even if it resulted in the loss of some jobs and building material?	56	39	9.1 ($P \leq .0001$)
A large coastal city has an unemployment problem. A major manufacturer want to build a new plant on a marsh it owns which could employ 1,000 people, but conservationists claim this will destroy land needed by a rare bird. Do you agree that this plant should be built, even if it endangers the bird species?	38	55	9.1 ($P \leq .0001$)

Table 10. Endangered Species Scale (Mean Scores) by Selected Demographic Groups: 1978 National Sample†

Demographic Groups (High)	Mean Score (Scale Max. = 56)
Students (Largely College)	28.4
Non-Ph.D. Graduate	28.4
18 - 25 Years Old	28.1
Single	27.8
1 Million+ Population	27.4
Alaska	26.7
Demographic Group	
General Population	24.8
56-65 Years Old	22.8
Southern Region	22.8
Less than 500 Population	22.4
Farming	22.1
6th - 8th Grade Education	21.6
75+ Years Old	20.7

†All differences between high and low groups and between these groups and the General Population score were significant at $P \leq .001$ according to analysis of variance results

Table 11. General Public and Livestock Producer Attitudes Toward Different Methods of Coyote Control

Question 1. Shoot or trap as many coyotes as possible.
Question 2. Poisoning, because it is the least expensive solution even though other animals may be killed.
Question 3. Whenever possible, hunt only individual coyotes known to have killed livestock.
Question 4. Capture and relocate coyotes away from sheep even though this is a very expensive solution.

		% Approved‡			
Group	**# Polled**	**Question 1**	**Question 2**	**Question 3**	**Question 4**
General Public					
Informed	548	38‡	8	71	67
Uninformed	1833	44‡	10	77	69
Sheep Producers	134	96	75	43	17
Cattlemen	124	94	70	52	10
All Groups, $(\chi)^2$		778.12	964.64	195.95	650.55
$(\chi)^2$ P Value		.0001	.0001	.0001	.0001

† In all cases, % disapproved can be obtained by subtracting from 100

‡ The χ^2 value for informed versus uninformed public was 56.61 and it had a P value of less than 0.0001

Table 12. Attitudes toward Hunting

Question: Of the following reasons for hunting, which do you approve of or oppose?

Reason	# Polled	% Approve Strong	% Approve Moderate	% Approve Slight	% Disapprove Slight	% Disapprove Moderate	% Disapprove Strong
Traditional native hunting (e.g. by Eskimos and Indians)	2379	16.2	47.5 (82)*	18.4	5.9	6.8 (15)	2.1
Hunting game mammals for recreation and sport	2417	4.4	18.6 (37)	13.6	10.9	27.3 (62)	23.6
Hunting waterfowl for recreation and sport†	2425	4.6	19.1 (40)	15.8	11.9	25.9 (59)	21.4
Hunting for meat	2429	22.1	46.5 (85)	16.6	5.5	5.1 (14)	3.1
Hunting for recreation and meat‡	2417	9.2	31.7 (64)	23.3	11.7	13.9 (34)	8.5
Hunting for a trophy	2412	2.0	7.8 (18)	8.4	9.4	26.7 (80)	44.1

* Number in parentheses ( ) is total of approve or disapprove

† Difference between approve and disapprove, $Z \leq 9.81$, P .0001

‡ Difference between approve and disapprove, $Z \leq 15.07$, P .0001

Table 13. Attitudes of General Public and Trappers Toward the Use of Steel Traps

Statement: I see nothing wrong with using steel traps to capture wild animals.

Group†	# Polled	% Agree Strong	% Agree Moderate	% Agree Slight	% Disagree Slight	% Disagree Moderate	% Disagree Strong
Informed Public	929	3.9	11.6 (20)‡	4.9	8.0	23.4 (79)	47.1
Uninformed Public	841	1.2	10.4 (19)	7.5	11.6	32.6 (74)	30.2
Trappers	171	81.9	12.9 (96)	1.2	2.9	0.6 (4)	0.6

† The χ^2 value is 676.98 ($P < .001$) for the differences between the general public and the trappers.

‡ Number in parentheses ( ) is total of agree or disagree.

Table 14. Public Attitudes Toward Wildlife Habitat Protection

Question	% Agree	% Disagree	Z Values
Natural resources must be developed even if the loss of wilderness results in much smaller wildlife populations.	44	51	3.28 ($P = 0.001$)
I approve of building on marshes that ducks and other nonendangered wildlife use if the marshes are needed for housing development.	39	57	8.94 ($P \leq 0.0001$)
Cutting trees for lumber and paper should be done in ways that help wildlife even if this results in higher timber prices.	76	20	28.22 ($P \leq 0.0001$)
Cattle and sheep grazing should be limited on publicly owned lands if it destroys plants needed by wildlife, even though this may result in higher meat costs.	60	34	13.02 ($P \leq 0.0001$)

TABLE I — Scale Mean Scores by Selected Animal Activity Groups: 1978 National Sample

	NAT	ECO	HUM	MOR	SCI	UTI	DOM	NEG
Max. Poss. Score†	**16**	**11**	**11**	**20**	**13**	**27**	**18**	**17**
General Population	3.1	3.1	4.0	5.5	0.9	5.3	2.0	4.4
Anti-Hunters	3.4	3.2	4.6	7.9	1.0	4.4	1.2	4.1
Backpackers	5.4	4.5	4.4	7.0	1.6	3.7	2.3	2.7
Birdwatchers	6.3	5.4	3.7	5.5	2.0	3.7	2.6	2.6
Env. Protect. Org. Memb.	6.5	7.7	4.8	9.6	1.9	1.6	1.5	1.5
Fishermen	4.0	3.6	4.1	4.4	1.0	5.4	3.0	3.6
Gen. Conserv. Org. Memb.	4.6	4.5	4.1	6.3	1.6	4.0	2.2	3.1
Humane Org. Memb.	5.6	5.1	6.1	9.5	1.8	3.0	0.9	2.7
Meat Hunters	4.1	3.9	4.0	4.2	1.0	5.6	3.3	3.2
Livestock Raisers	3.2	3.2	3.2	4.5	1.0	7.3	2.7	4.5
Nature Hunters	8.5	5.7	3.9	4.8	1.5	3.8	3.8	2.9
Scientific Study	5.7	5.3	4.5	8.0	2.7	3.3	1.8	2.2
Sport-Rec. Hunters	3.8	3.8	3.8	2.9	1.2	5.4	4.1	3.4
Sportsmen Org. Memb.	5.7	5.4	3.8	4.3	1.4	4.8	4.1	2.7
Wildlf. Protect. Org. Memb.	5.8	6.3	4.4	7.7	2.2	2.9	1.7	2.7
Zoo Visitors	4.4	3.6	4.8	7.1	1.2	4.0	1.5	3.4
1978 Mail Sample								
Cattlemen	3.9	5.2	3.2	1.3	0.9	13.1	5.1	3.8
Natl. Trappers	9.6	7.3	4.0	2.8	1.8	3.4	8.5	2.1
Sheep Producers	3.7	4.5	3.3	2.0	1.08	12.8	4.7	3.9

† The score maxima for each attitude varies because there was a different number of questions for each attitude with different scorin For example, there were eight questions for the **Naturalistic** attitude with a score of either 2 or 0 for three questions and scores of 2,1 or for the other five. The number of questions for the other attitudes are (in the order listed in the table) 4, 5, 10, 6, 13, 8 and 8, respectivel

TABLE II — Demographic Groups (selected) and Mean Scores for Different Attitudes.

	NAT	ECO	HUM	MOR	SCI	UTI	DOM	NEG
Max. Poss. Score	**16**	**11**	**11**	**20**	**13**	**27**	**18**	**17**
General Population	3.1	3.1	4.0	5.5	0.9	5.3	2.0	4.4
Regions								
Alaska	4.6	4.4	3.7	4.5	1.3	4.1	2.4	2.4
North Central	*	*	*	*	*	*	*	*
North East	*	*	*	*	*	*	*	*
Pacific	3.6	3.6	4.4	7.5	*	*	1.5	*
Rocky Mountain	*	*	*	*	*	*	2.3	*
Southern	*	*	3.6	4.5	*	6.4	2.3	*
General Groups								
Male	3.4	3.4	3.6	4.7	*	*	2.6	*
Female	*	*	4.3	6.0	*	*	1.5	*
Black	2.1	2.4	3.7	*	*	6.4	2.5	5.6
White	*	*	*	*	*	*	*	*
Married	*	*	*	*	*	*	*	*
Single	3.6	*	4.3	6.1	1.3	4.1	*	*
Never Religious Service	3.9	3.7	4.3	6.7	1.2	4.1	*	*
1 Week Religious Service	*	2.8	3.5	*	*	5.9	*	*
Education								
<6th Grade	1.3	2.3	2.4	3.6	0.4	6.9	2.6	6.4
6th-8th Grade	2.1	2.6	3.4	4.7	0.6	7.1	2.4	5.8
9th-12th Grade	2.4	2.5	*	*	0.6	6.1	*	5.1
Student	4.0	3.6	4.4	6.7	1.6	3.9	1.7	3.3
Non-PhD. Graduate	4.5	4.5	*	6.8	1.7	4.2	*	3.0
PhD.	*	5.3	4.6	7.3	1.9	3.7	1.5	2.3
Employment								
Unemployed	2.4	2.7	*	*	*	*	*	*
Retired	2.5	*	3.7	*	*	6.3	1.8	5.3
Vocational	2.7	2.7	3.7	*	*	6.4	*	5.3
Professional	3.7	3.6	*	6.2	1.2	4.6	1.7	*
Unskilled	*	2.8	*	4.6	*	*	2.5	*
Blue Collar	2.7	2.8	*	*	*	*	*	*
Service	2.6	2.8	*	*	*	*	*	*
Farming	2.4	2.7	3.1	3.7	*	8.5	2.7	5.3
Age								
18-25 Years Old	3.4	*	4.8	6.2	1.2	4.1	*	3.5
26-35 Years Old	*	3.4	*	6.1	1.2	4.2	1.8	*
56-65 Years Old	*	2.8	3.7	*	0.6	6.4	*	*
66-75 Years Old	2.5	2.6	3.4	4.7	0.6	7.0	*	5.3
75+ Years Old	2.2	2.6	3.2	*	0.4	7.1	*	6.0

TABLE II (Continued)

	NAT	ECO	HUM	MOR	SCI	UTI	DOM	NEG
Income								
<$5,000	2.6	2.7	3.7	*	0.7	6.1	2.3	5.4
$15,000-14,999	3.4	*	*	6.0	*	4.6	*	*
$25,000-34,999	3.6	3.5	4.5	*	*	*	*	*
$50,000-99,999	*	3.7	*	4.7	*	*	2.6	3.5
Population - Childhood Community								
<500	*	2.8	3.4	4.0	0.7	6.4	2.4	*
25,000-49,999	3.5	3.4	*	6.7	*	4.6	1.7	*
250,000-999,999	3.4	3.4	4.3	6.0	1.2	*	*	*
1 Million +	*	*	*	6.4	*	4.6	1.8	*
Population — Present Community								
<500	*	*	3.2	3.3	*	6.3	2.5	*
25,000-49,999	3.6	3.4	4.4	6.1	1.2	4.7	*	*
250,000-999,999			4.3	*	*	*	1.8	
1 Million+	*	*	*	6.3	*	*	*	*

* Mean Scores are the same (*i.e.* do not differ significantly) as those reported for the General Population

TABLE III — Analysis of Variance of Selected Demographic Variables by Attitude Scales*

Variable	F Values							
	NAT	ECO	HUM	MOR	SCI	UTI	DOM	NEG
Age	9.64†	2.53‡	11.31†	3.35‡	15.69†	24.95†	0.99	15.9
Population of Present Residence	1.08	0.56	0.74	2.47‡	0.91	1.70	1.68	2.4
Region	5.03†	3.42†	4.06†	12.50†	0.56	10.01†	6.98†	6.4
Education	12.03†	18.37†	0.56	4.82†	20.03†	4.49†	2.71‡	13.2
Occupation	0.73	1.72	1.79	1.84	0.57	3.28†	1.88	0.6
Religiosity	4.97†	4.41†	5.34†	6.38†	1.06	5.09†	3.62†	2.4
Income	3.69†	1.33	5.56†	1.59	0.34	3.92†	0.84	5.4
Marital Status	0.69	0.32	0.63	1.81	6.12†	5.55†	0.27	1.7
Race	15.13†	11.45†	2.39	0.94	0.60	11.54†	6.10†	23.0
Sex	23.16†	26.90†	63.12†	63.18†	1.52	20.76†	183.93†	128.9

* Only main effect F values and significance levels are indicated. Two analysis of variance tests were performed. The first included main effects age, population of present residence, region, education, occupation, and, as covariates attendance at religious servi (religiosity), income, marital status, race and sex. The second run included as main effects religiosity, income, marital status, race & sex, and, as covariates age, population of present residence and education. Occupation and region could not be included covariates in the second analysis due to their nonlinear character.

† F value has significance of less than 0.01

‡ F value has significance of less than 0.05

TABLE IV — Multiple Classification Analysis of Selected Demographic Variables for the Naturalistic, Ecologistic, Humanistic and Moralistic scales.

(See Table III for note on performance of the analysis.)

Naturalistic (Max Score = 16)

Group	Deviation†
Graduate Education	1.13
Alaska	0.85
18-25 Years Old	0.52
26-35 Years Old	0.36
College Education	0.36
Pacific Coast	0.31
Rarely/Never attend Religious Services	0.31
Clerical Occupation	-0.44
76+ Years Old	-0.49
56-75 Years Old	-0.54
9-11th Grade Education	-0.54
Less than 8th Grade education	-0.61
Black	-0.87

Ecologistic (Max Score = 11)

Group	Deviation†
Graduate Education	1.28
Alaska	0.94
Prof./Manag. Occ.	0.31
Rarely/Never Attend Religious Service	0.27
Male	0.27
500-1,999 Pop.	0.24
56-75 Years Old	-0.29
Unskilled Blue Collar	-0.32
Less than 8th Grade Education	-0.35
9-11th Grade Education	-0.58
Black	-0.62

Humanistic (Max Score = 11)

Group	Deviation†
18-25 Years Old	0.71
$20,000-34,999 Income	0.36
Female	0.33
Rarely/Never Attend Religious Service	0.31
Pacific Coast	0.27
Less than 500 Pop. -0.42	South
Male	-0.45
Alaska	-0.58
76+ Years Old	-0.67
Farmers	-0.90
Less than 500 Pop.	-1.50

Moralistic (Max Poss. Score = 20)

Group	Deviation†
Pacific Coast	1.59
Clerical Workers	1.37
Graduate Education	1.32
Female	0.64
Rarely/Never Attend Religious Service	0.61
26-34 Years Old	0.49
18-25 Years Old	0.44
-0.80	
500-1,999 Pop.	-0.83
Male	-0.86
Farmers	-0.94
Alaska	-1.38

†All deviations listed above are significant. The positive deviations indicate greater than average prevalence of the attitude, and negative deviations lower than average prevalence of the attitude.

TABLE V — Multiple Classification Analysis of Selected Demographic Variables for the Scientistic, Utilitarian, Dominionistic, and Negativistic Scales.

(See Table III for a note on performance of the analysis.)

Scientistic (Max. Poss. Score = 13)

Group	Deviation†
Graduate Education	0.83
18-25 Years Old	0.30
26-35 Years Old	0.28
Single	0.22
College Education	0.17
Alaska	0.10
High School Vocat. Education	-0.19
Less than 8th Grade Education	-0.21
9th-11th Grade Education	-0.22
56-75 Years Old	-0.30
76 + Years Old	-0.38

Dominionistic (Max. Poss. Score = 18)

Group	Deviation†
Male	0.68
Farmers	0.66
Alaska	0.43
Rocky Mt. States	0.37
$35,000 + Income	0.23
Rarely Never attend Religious Services	-0.21
Clerical Workers	-0.36
Graduate Education	-0.45
Female	-0.51
Pacific Coast	-0.55

Utilitarian (Max. Poss. Score = 27)

Group	Deviation†
Farmers	2.11
76 + Years Old	1.43
56-75 Years Old	1.15
Black	1.13
South	0.88
1 Million + Pop.	-0.45
Single	-0.61
Alaska	-0.70
Graduate Education	-0.85
26-36 Years Old	-0.88
18-25 Years Old	-1.14

Negativistic (Max. Poss. Score = 17)

Group	Deviation†
Black	1.08
Less than 8th Grade Education	0.95
76 + Years Old	0.74
Female	0.51
56-75 Years Old	0.50
Less than 500 Pop.	-0.59
Male	-0.68
18-25 Years Old	-0.69
Graduate Education	-0.99
Alaska	-1.16

† All deviations listed above are significant. The positive deviations indicate greater than average prevalence of the attitude, and negative deviations lower than average prevalence of the attitude.

REFERENCES

Ehrenfeld, D.W. 1970. *Biological conservation*, New York, N.Y.: Holt, Rinehart, and Winston.

Guggisberg, C.A.W. 1970. *Man and wildlife*, New York, N.Y.: Arco Publishing Company.

Kellert, S.R. 1976. *Perceptions of animals in American society*. Transactions of the 41st North American Wildlife and Natural Resources Conference, Wildlife Management Office, Washington, D.C., pp. 533–46.

Kellert, S.R. 1978. *Policy implications of a national study of American attitudes and behavioral relations to animals*. U.S. Fish and Wildlife Service, U.S. Department of the Interior, Stock Number 024-101-00482-7, U.S. Government Printing Office, Washington, D.C.

Kellert, S.R. 1979a. *Public attitudes toward critical wildlife and natural habitat issues: Phase I*, U.S. Fish and Wildlife Service, U.S. Department of the Interior, Washington, D.C.

Kellert, S.R. 1979b. Contemporary values of wildlife in American society. *Methods of assessing and categorizing values of wildlife*. Rocky Mountain Forest and Range Experiment Station, (In press).

Ziswiler, V. 1967. *Extinct and vanishing animals*. London, U.K.: The English Universities Press.

INSTRUCTIONS TO AUTHORS

Manuscripts: Footnotes, references, tables, and figure legends are to be typewritten, double-spaced on 8½ x 11 inch bond paper leaving generous margins. Manuscripts must be in English using the preferred spelling in the Webster's Third International Dictionary. Submit original and two (2) copies.

Manuscript organization: Title page (p. 1) containing title of the manuscript, author(s) affiliation, present address wherever proofs should be sent; Text (beginning p. 2), with introduction, methods, procedures, results, discussion, conclusion, acknowledgments, references, tables, and figure legends. Special instructions for the copy editor or printer should be affixed to the original copy.

Abbreviations and units: Standard dictionary abbreviations are generally accepted. Other abbreviations should be explained when first mentioned. SI units are preferred.

References: The Author-Date system, not a numbering system, should be used for the citation of references in the text, e.g., Jones (1977) or (Jones and Smith 1977) or (Jones et.al. 1977) for more than three authors of one citation. When citing the authors of such papers in the reference list, *all* authors must be listed for citations using et.al. in the text. Where more than one paper by the same author (s) has appeared in one year, the reference should be distinguished by "a," "b," "c," etc. (e.g. 1971a). The list of references should be arranged alphabetically by authors' last names, and chronologically per author. Titles: Journals should be abbreviated in accordance with the *Chemical Abstract Service Source Index.* References to books/monographs should include editors, edition/volume number, publisher, city, and state/country where published and relevant page numbers. A paper in press may be referenced if it has been accepted for publication. References to personal communications and unpublished work are permitted in the text only.

sample references: (in accordance with the University of Chicago, *A Manual of Style.*)

Smith, J. 1970. The effect of stress in swine on meat quality. *J. Appl. Ethol.* 5:125-7.

Smith, J. and Jones, S. 1978. *Animals and environment.* 2nd ed. New York:Academic Press.

Tables: These should be concise and double-spaced throughout.

Figures: Submit three sets of glossy prints (no negatives) with identifying arrows and letters contrasting sharply with the background. Indicate on the back the author's name, figure number, and "top."

Figure legends: Captions should contain sufficient information allowing the figures to be clearly understood without reference to the text.

Review of manuscripts: All manuscripts submitted will be subjected to prior review and approval by the Manuscript Review Committee.

GPSR Compliance
The European Union's (EU) General Product Safety Regulation (GPSR) is a set of rules that requires consumer products to be safe and our obligations to ensure this.

If you have any concerns about our products, you can contact us on

ProductSafety@springernature.com

In case Publisher is established outside the EU, the EU authorized representative is:

Springer Nature Customer Service Center GmbH
Europaplatz 3
69115 Heidelberg, Germany

www.ingramcontent.com/pod-product-compliance
Ingram Content Group UK Ltd.
Pitfield, Milton Keynes, MK11 3LW, UK
UKHW020136160926
475607UK00003B/81
9780898386998